The Social Production of Crisis

The Social Production of Crisis

Blood, Politics, and Death in France and the United States

CONSTANCE A. NATHANSON
AND HENRI BERGERON

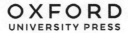

OXFORD
UNIVERSITY PRESS

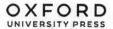

OXFORD
UNIVERSITY PRESS

Oxford University Press is a department of the University of Oxford. It furthers
the University's objective of excellence in research, scholarship, and education
by publishing worldwide. Oxford is a registered trade mark of Oxford University
Press in the UK and certain other countries.

Published in the United States of America by Oxford University Press
198 Madison Avenue, New York, NY 10016, United States of America.

CIP data is on file at the Library of Congress
ISBN 978-0-19-768248-7

DOI: 10.1093/oso/9780197682487.001.0001

Printed by Integrated Books International, United States of America

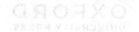

For Ronald Bayer and Didier Tabuteau
Mentors and Pioneers

Preface

Doing full justice to the origins of this book would require digging deep into the early life of its first author, Connie Nathanson, growing up in Chicago and learning at her mother's knee—or, more likely, on her lap—that there was more than one language in the world and that language was—*French*. Fast forward to the early 2000s and a seminar in New York City by William Dab, a sometime counselor to France's minister of health. Throughout a long career at the intersection of sociology and public health, France had never lost its grip on Nathanson's imagination, and she was then deep in a project comparing public health dramas in four countries, including France and the United States, where France was coming off as a distinct laggard in the public health arena (Nathanson 2007). Imagine her surprise and excitement as Dab described the recent passage of a new public health law! Further investigation revealed a marked and very recent revival of attention to public health in France originating with a major political crisis around the "discovery" of HIV-contaminated blood as a public problem in the early 1990s. Nathanson was off and running. Very quickly, through the good offices of Columbia University's Alliance Program, she found a magnificent partner in Henri Bergeron, and they have worked closely together ever since. It was only after several years of research that we came to realize the potential value of a comparison with the United States, and this delay partially accounts for what may seem to some readers a disproportionate emphasis on France. Our only excuse is that the French story is disproportionately fascinating.

We were incredibly lucky that the onsite archival work for this project as well as oral history interviews with French actors in the blood drama were completed in February 2020 just before COVID-19 shut archives and libraries down and made overseas travel impossible. We were also incredibly lucky to have a consummate expert in internet sleuthing, Ian Bradley-Perrin, join our team in late 2019. A French-speaking graduate student in history, Ian found online treasure suspected, unsuspected, and hidden, enriching our data beyond anything we could have done without him. Archival and online sources are listed in Appendix C.

This project has accumulated many debts over its long gestation, but our most powerful obligation is to Didier Tabuteau who not only gave us his unflagging interest and support but also made possible our access to key documents in France's National Archives that would normally have been closed to scholars. We owe special debts of gratitude to Sophie Chauveau who shared with us her postdoctoral thesis, "From the Gift to the Market," on the long history of blood in France and to Jessie Saul for sharing her doctoral dissertation, the first to carry out a direct comparison of France with the United States. Colleagues at Columbia University in New York and at Sciences Po in Paris—Patrick Castel, Gil Eyal, Jennifer Hirsch, Kim Hopper, Etienne Nouguez, Kavita Sivaramakrishnan—read and commented on various drafts or simply listened to our ideas, each contributing immeasurably to the final product. Others who read papers drawn from this project and encouraged us on the way include Julia Adams, Ashley Fox, and Gowri Vijayakumar. We benefited as well from critical intellectual support for research and writing at the intersection of history, sociology, and policy from Columbia's Center for the History & Ethics of Public Health and the Columbia Population Research Center (CPRC), the Chaire Santé at Sciences Po and the Laboratoire interdisciplinaire d'évaluation des politiques publiques (LIEPP) in Paris. We would like to offer special thanks to Sébastien Plouhinec, then at Sciences Po, who with warmth and enthusiasm went beyond the call of duty in easing Nathanson's first steps in this project and to Ronald Bayer, whose unfailing instinct for a good story paved the way. Actors in the drama of contaminated blood both in France and the United States contributed invaluable experience and insights in the form of extended interviews; they also have our deepest thanks.

Research for this book drew on many and disparate archival resources and consequently on the time and talents of the individuals—some of whose names we know and some we do not—who manage those resources. We owe a special debt of gratitude to Hervé Lemoine, director of the French National Archives during the period of our research, and to the invariably helpful staff at each of its two sites, Fontainebleau and Pierre-Fitte, where we spent long hours and asked many questions. We would like to thank Kimberly Springer, Curator for Oral History at Columbia; Guy Hall at the National Archives in Atlanta; Mary E. Hilpertshauser, Manager of Historic Collections at the David J. Sencer CDC Museum; Janice Goldblum at the National Academy of Sciences; and Vincent Szukala, Assistant Archivist at the French Cour des comptes all of whom were extraordinarily helpful in pointing us in the right directions and retrieving (apparently) inaccessible items. We are equally grateful to the many other archivists whose collections (listed in Appendix C) we drew on in France and the United States.

Research and writing for this book was supported by the Columbia Alliance Program, the National Library of Medicine, the National Science Foundation, and the John Simon Guggenheim Foundation. Cross-national projects are complicated and expensive, and we are immeasurably thankful to each of these institutions for the support that made this book possible.

Finally, we would like to thank Oxford University Press and, in particular, James Cook for his patience over the many years it took to bring this book to fruition.

Contents

Contents

1

Introduction

This is the tale of two countries' struggle with HIV contamination of the blood supply in the last decades of the twentieth century, dramatic and with continuing resonance in France, while largely forgotten in the United States. "Everything began with AIDS and the affair of the tainted blood," wrote François Grémy, among the deans of French public health. "Like a clap of thunder in the sky of good health and medical progress, the entire society found itself caught in the winds of panic, traumatized, disoriented in relation to its most constant beacons" (2004:195).

Here we tell the story of how and why this health catastrophe became a political crisis in France and in the United States a mere sideshow to the vast drama that was AIDS. But our aims go beyond telling a good story. Our narrative is structured as a case comparison in the expectation that attention to the details of historical events of a similar kind but with different outcomes will contribute to the understanding of larger social processes—in this instance, the social production of political crisis.

We begin with a brief foreshadowing of these larger processes, to be examined and illustrated more fully in the chapters that follow. Grounded in our data—the French and American blood stories—and in multiple overlapping strands of sociological theory, we argue that the social production of political crisis happens on three levels: first, underlying contradictions in the institutional logics (beliefs and practices) that animate an important "field" of action in the polity (see, e.g., Seo and Creed 2002, Clemens and Cook 1999, Thornton et al. 2012); second, a process of "strategic mobilization" that renders those contradictions visible in the public sphere (see, e.g., Morris 1993, Fligstein and McAdam 2012, Alexander 2018, 2019); and third, an array of cultural beliefs (schemas, symbolic constructions) that frames those contradictions as immoral and unacceptable (see, e.g., Sewell 1992, 1996).[1] Contradiction in the logics applied to human blood—as gift or

---

[1] The nearest approximation to our theory of the social production of crisis is Alexander's theory of "societalization" as described in his 2019 book, *What Makes a Social Crisis? The Societalization*

The Social Production of Crisis. Constance A. Nathanson and Henri Bergeron, Oxford University Press.
© Oxford University Press 2023. DOI: 10.1093/oso/9780197682487.003.0001

commodity—emerged almost simultaneously with recognition of its therapeutic potential. The HIV/blood affair triggered strategic mobilization in response to those contradictions, their denunciation—in France but not in the United States—as immoral and unacceptable and—again in France but not in the United States—a crisis of political legitimacy.

Epidemics of infectious disease are at one and the same time patterned—dramas with first and (at least historically) final acts—and unique in each society's response (Rosenberg 1989). It is in this uniqueness that the fascination—and importance—of case comparison resides. The traditional first act, captured by Camus in the opening pages of *The Plague*, is one not so much of denial but disbelief: "So long as each individual doctor had come across only two or three cases, no one had thought of taking action . . . the public mustn't be alarmed" (Camus [1948] 1991:35).[2] Consistent with this pattern, the initial responses of both French and American blood bankers to early alarms about HIV contamination of the blood supply combined disbelief, uncertainty, and denial. Once government officials and politicians became involved, however, responses sharply diverged. Close attention to when, how, and why they diverged illuminates the many ways that country-specific institutions and cultures shape the politics of epidemic disease.

The clap of thunder that triggered the HIV/blood crisis was a magazine article: "The Report That Accuses the National Blood Transfusion Center"—its title evoking Zola's famous "*J'accuse*" of 1898 attacking the French government's actions in the Dreyfus affair. Written by a physician turned medical journalist, the article was published on April 25, 1991, in a bi-weekly news magazine *L'Événement du jeudi* (Casteret 1991).[3] Its centerpiece was the verbatim record (visibly stamped "confidential") of a meeting on May 29, 1985, of the director and senior medical staff of the Centre National de Transfusion Sanguine (CNTS).[4] The record made clear that this group of elite blood bankers had known in the spring of 1985 that blood

---

of Social Problems. Theories of crisis have an important intellectual history, which is beyond our present scope.

[2] For a current instance of this pattern, see Bergeron et al. *Covid-19: Une crise organisationnelle* (Paris: Presses de la Fondation Nationale des Sciences Politiques, 2020).

[3] There is virtual unanimity among French scholars, politicians, and journalists (Chauveau 2011, Fillion 2009, Tabuteau 2006, Nau 2011, personal communication) in attributing the "clap of thunder" to Casteret's article.

[4] "National Blood Transfusion Center" is misleading. The Centre National de Transfusion Sanguine (CNTS) was a large regional blood bank centered in Paris, one of seven regional banks. It had specialized functions assigned by the Ministry of Health, but it was not a "national" blood bank. Whether it was an agency of the government was highly contested.

used in the CNTS's manufacture of blood products for hemophiliacs was HIV contaminated, that these physicians made a conscious decision not to withdraw those products, and that this decision was driven at least in part by financial considerations.[5] This revelation—the invasion of the market into the sacred domain of blood—rapidly became the focal point of the drama that was to follow, transforming the blood affair in France from "*fatalité*" to "*scandale*" and, simultaneously, into a symbol of government betrayal of its citizens' trust.[6]

From the date of Casteret's revelation, events in France rapidly descended into political crisis. A media storm ensued; the head of the CNTS resigned within little over a month and was indicted; and the government acknowledged "serious errors" and called for an investigation. In a dramatic trial extending over the summer months of 1992 and attracting breathless media coverage as well as protests from Act Up-Paris on behalf of HIV-infected hemophiliacs, blood bankers and government health officials were tried, three (out of four) were convicted, and one was ultimately imprisoned. The "*affair du sang*" has become a key point of reference in French historical, political, and public health analyses of the 1980s, 1990s, and beyond. Ripples from its impact continue to this day.

HIV contamination of the blood supply happened in all industrialized countries in the early 1980s. Both in France and in the United States the scope of the ensuing medical catastrophe was almost unimaginable in the numbers infected and in mortality. In both countries, slightly more than 50% of the total hemophilia population was infected (up to 90% of severe hemophiliacs), amounting to over 8,000 people in the United States and approximately 1,200 in France.[7] Depending on population estimates, between 25% and 40% of hemophiliacs in the United States would eventually die of AIDS. An estimated 12,000 transfusion recipients were infected in the ed States and close to 2,000 in France. The bulk of HIV infections occurred

---

[5] Hemophilia is a relatively rare inherited sex-linked disorder that interferes with blood clotting. Females carry the hemophilia gene, but the disease manifests itself almost entirely in males.

[6] Organization of French blood services is fully described in Chapter 2. Contestation notwithstanding, CNTS was *not* in fact a government agency in the period of which we speak. Along with all French blood banks, it was financed and operated independently with minimal government oversight. Government control of the blood supply was precipitated by the blood crisis (Bergeron and Nathanson 2012, Nathanson and Bergeron 2017). In the process of mobilization on behalf of hemophiliacs, CNTS was actively *transformed* into a symbol of government malfeasance.

[7] In the absence of systematic surveillance at the time, estimates of the total number of hemophiliacs in each country are approximate. Numbers infected and mortality are reasonably reliable, based on national statistics.

before 1985 when measures to protect the blood supply—blood donor screening, blood testing, and heat treatment (virus inactivation) of blood products intended for hemophiliacs—were put in place.

Both countries confronted the same scientific uncertainties on the etiology and course of the AIDS epidemic, and there was marked overlap in key actors (blood bankers, government health officials, legislators, militant hemophiliacs) and, retrospectively, in the identification of institutional failures. Nevertheless, the two countries sharply diverged in how this catastrophe was framed retrospectively and in modes of response. In France, recognition of a public health catastrophe produced a political crisis reaching the highest levels of government. In the United States, with an AIDS case rate among hemophiliacs double the rate in France, there was no comparable political crisis. The empirical questions we address in this book are straightforward: Why was there a political crisis in France and why in the United States did the deaths of up to half a community create barely a ripple?

Assertions about "crisis" and "political crisis" beg the questions of how we define these concepts and what are the grounds for our claim that there was a "political crisis" in one country and not in the other. We return to those questions below, but first we address the prior question of why revisit the HIV/blood story at all. There already exists a substantial literature on each country's separate experience (far more extensive in France than in the United States),[8] and a few comparative studies that include France and the United States among other Western countries.[9] Nevertheless, there is no published work with the explicit aim of comparing the French experience of the HIV/blood affair with that of the United States. This comparison is important for three reasons. First, it presents a unique opportunity to unravel the social and institutional processes that underlie the production of political crisis. Second, the contrasting patterns of social mobilization, litigation, and state action between the two countries are in many respects

[8] France: Casteret 1992, Chauveau 2007, 2011, Fillion 2009, Girard 1998, Grémy 2004, Hermitte 1996, Marchetti 2010, Morelle 1996, Sourdille and Huriet 1992, Steffen 1999, Roux 1995, Tabuteau 2006; United States: Bayer 1999, Healy 2006, Institute of Medicine 1995, Lederer 2008, Resnik 1999, Shilts 1987, Siplon 2002.

[9] Feldman 2000, Feldman and Bayer 1999, Glied 1996, Trebilcock et al. 1996, Saul 2004. Jessie Saul's unpublished doctoral dissertation, "The Tainted Gift: A Comparative Study of the Culture and Politics of the Contamination of the Blood Supply with the AIDS Virus in France and the United States," is the only one of these works that directly addresses the question, why was there a blood "scandal" in France and not the United States. However, in answering this question Saul focuses heavily on media framing of events in the two countries in the period 1985–1991, largely omitting the historical, political, institutional, and organizational contexts in which these framings were embedded and through which they must be understood.

counterintuitive, belying the image of France as a closed state impervious to social movement mobilization and court action (Kitschelt 1986). Third, this book contributes to knowledge of how and why questions of scientific governance are answered differently in France than in the United States. For example, the political crisis that attended the French public's discovery of HIV contamination of the blood supply played a key role in French adoption of the "precautionary principle" in approaching scientific and health risks (Tabuteau 2006), a role that has been largely ignored in earlier work on the spread of this principle in Europe (see, e.g., Jasanoff 2005, Vogel 2012).[10]

More broadly, in the larger sweep of the AIDS narrative, the blood story and its victims have been easy for AIDS scholars in the United States to disregard and forget. Compared with sex and drugs, blood and blood transfusion may have appeared as morally neutral modes of HIV transmission. They did not carry the charge of wicked and disreputable acts or the opportunity to fight inequality and discrimination that animated the larger AIDS narrative and excited its chroniclers.[11] In this vast literature, hemophiliacs and random hospital patients who had the misfortune to need blood at the wrong moment in history were often treated as collateral damage—accident victims who got in the way of a steamroller directed elsewhere, not intended for them, and of correspondingly less interest to historians and social scientists.[12] With this book, we aim to bring this dramatic story of blood, politics, and death out of the shadows.

Theorizing Crises

We define "crises" as widely recognized and consequential ruptures in human affairs. This definition is very close to what Sahlins (1985) and Sewell (1996) label "events"; our use of "crisis" is intended to avoid confusion with routine events on the order of weddings, funerals, and theater first nights.

[10] This project also takes advantage of unique sources of data: French health cabinet internal documents for the period 1988–2003 normally unavailable for forty years after their original deposit with the French national archives; recently (2016) released oral history interviews with CDC professional staff closely involved with the early days of the AIDS epidemic; just released archives of Randy Shilts deposited with the San Francisco Public Library relevant to the early days of AIDS in France, including interviews with the research team that discovered the HIV virus. .

[11] In fact, hemophiliacs in the United States were often categorized with homosexuals and suffered equivalent stigma and discrimination (Davidson 2008, IOM 1995).

[12] Baldwin's treatment of hemophiliacs and the transfused in his comprehensive comparative history of AIDS is fairly typical (Baldwin 2005).

Sewell's exemplary—and telling—event (crisis) is the taking of the Bastille on July 14, 1789, that launched the French Revolution. But to become "widely recognized," even the storming of the Bastille demanded interpretation. Why were not the bloody occurrences of that day dismissed as yet one more instance of mob rule in the notoriously unruly city of Paris? Labeling an occurrence as a crisis is not given by the circumstances at hand. It is an *attribution of meaning* by interested actors who have a stake in the production of crisis and in its outcome. Even natural disasters—earthquakes and floods (think Katrina)—do not invariably speak for themselves. As eloquently put by Senator Mike De Wine (R-OH) in the course of a congressional hearing on compensation for hemophiliacs in the United States, "bad things happen to good people all the time." Rarely do these bad things enter the public sphere and become occasions for public drama and moral outrage as they did in France during the early 1990s.

Social Production of Crisis

This book is a series of overlapping, more or less chronologically organized, stories about the social life of human blood in France and the United States.[13] The aim of these stories, however, is less historical than analytical—to understand how and why a contaminated blood crisis emerged in France through detailed comparison with the United States where there was no crisis: the *absence* of crisis is as important to this analysis as its presence. We will present a more fully developed conceptual framework in Chapter 9 (foreshadowed in our opening paragraphs), but our narratives are interspersed with theoretical reflection, and it will be well to say something here about the conceptual tools on which we rely: attributions of meaning; engaged actors; processes of mobilization; and the cultural, political, and institutional structures in and through which these processes played themselves out.

Attributions of meaning are central to contemporary sociological analyses of social problems: "Human problems do not spring up, full-blown and announced, into the consciousness of bystanders.[14] Even to recognize a

---

[13] We are indebted to Arjun Appadurai for his insight that "commodities, like persons, have social lives" (1986:3). Blood circulates not only within the body but also, like other objects of value, outside it in neighborhoods, communities, and states.

[14] "Sensemaking," as used by organizational theorists to describe peoples' ongoing "efforts to create order and make retrospective sense of what occurs," is a closely related concept (Weick 1993:635).

situation as painful requires a system [a cultural vocabulary] for categorizing and defining events" (Gusfield 1981:3). Social problems with the potential to become crises are *happenings interpreted* as painful, unexpected—outside the normal course of events, and significant. Attributions of meaning do not inhere in the happenings themselves. Further, the categories with which we make sense of happenings in the world *are social and cultural creations*, the product of "cultural schemas"—vocabularies of meaning and motive—particular to engaged actors. Crises are happenings interpreted, and interpretations vary. Blood—the centerpiece of our story—is fraught with meaning as sacred symbol, as technological marvel, as marketable commodity, and not only do these meanings vary among themselves but also their symbolic power in the cultural lexicons of our two countries differ markedly, as we shall see.

Equally important to our crisis narratives is the presence on the scene of interested and engaged actors. Meanings are created out of the categories available within a specific cultural context but "in action" they are "determined also as an 'interest,' which is the instrumental value to the acting subject" (Sahlins 1985:150). In other words, actors are not passive instruments for the deployment of preexisting cultural categories. They exercise *agency*, bending "categories to their own ends in the course of action" (Sewell 1996:203–4).[15] Interested actors who foresee gains in material or symbolic power from elevating a given painful condition out of obscurity into the public sphere have played an especially large part in the construction of public health problems (Nathanson 2007). Smoking, breast cancer, HIV/AIDS and, yes, contamination of the blood supply compete with each other on the public stage, and entrepreneurial groups and individuals "promote different problems or different ways of seeing the same problem" (Hilgartner and Bosk 1988:56) in an effort to dominate the current social problem discourse and appropriate to themselves what limited resources (of manpower, time, money, media space) may be available. On the surface, actors in the drama of contaminated blood were much the same in France and the United States: blood bankers, hemophiliacs and their physicians, gay groups, politicians, and health administrators, scientists, journalists, and lawyers and judges. Nor were their "interests" that far apart. Opportunities to act on

[15] Our use of "interests" is not limited to material or economic interests but includes being socially *invested* in a defined set of values or outcomes (see, e.g., Bourdieu 2014:272). Bourdieu's example is "feeling shattered when a public TV channel is abolished" (2014:272).

those interests were constrained both by the cultural categories at hand and by contingencies of relationship networks, institutional power, and historical and political context.

Interested actors must actively put their interests into play through *mobilization* in one form or another—engaging likeminded allies and supportive elites in identifying harms, assigning responsibility, and demanding change. McAdam and Scott have argued that "it is generally not the destabilizing events/processes themselves that set periods of field contention and change [i.e., crises] in motion. Rather it is a process of reactive *mobilization*" (2005:18). Mobilization, however, may occur in the interest of generating crisis as well as in response to it. Morris describes how civil rights movement actors in 1963 deliberately created a public crisis (large-scale economic and political protests) in Birmingham, Alabama, "of such magnitude that national and local white establishments would have no option but to capitulate" (1993:624; see also Fligstein and McAdam 2012:20). We will argue that something similar happened in France to produce the blood crisis. The United States has a storied tradition of social movement activism—and a comparable abundance of scholarship on the conditions for and processes of mobilization on which we will draw to understand how and why those processes played out so differently—and so unexpectedly—in French and American responses to the tragedy of HIV contaminated blood.

Among the keys to successful mobilization are *framing processes*: the "action-oriented sets of beliefs and meanings that inspire and legitimate [the movement's] activities and campaigns" (Benford and Snow 2000:614). Movement actors construct culturally resonant "beliefs and meanings" particular to their campaigns from the larger stock of schemas and ideologies available in their cultural settings. As Benford and Snow point out, this "cultural resource base" is not only the *source* for new collective action frames but also "the *lens* through which framings are interpreted and evaluated" (629, emphasis added). Lamont and Thévenot have proposed the concept of "national cultural repertoires of evaluation" to highlight the fact that "cultural tools . . . are unevenly available across situations and national contexts" (2000:1). In particular, as they emphasize repeatedly, "evaluations based on market performance are much more frequent in the United States than in France, while evaluations based on civic solidarity are more salient in France" (2001:2). Indeed, "business interests are understood [in France] to be incompatible with the general interest, both on political and moral grounds" (2001:13). These distinctions—and their consequences for mobilization and framing processes around the blood affair—are critical to our analysis of how and why political crisis was socially produced in France and not in the United States.

Finally, whether "happenings" are transformed into crises is highly contingent on the relationship structures and institutional, historical, and political contexts within which these events occur. As we noted above, the meanings and symbols deployed in crisis construction are available as resources to some actors and in some cultural contexts, but not in others. Incentives, power, and opportunities for effective mobilization are differentially distributed, dependent both on the immediate political context and on relatively stable dimensions of each country's cultural and political structures. Militant hemophiliacs in France, for example, were not forced to compete for attention in the public sphere with organized, active, and politically connected gay men already on the scene, as was the case in the United States. Unraveling how this difference—and other like contingencies—shaped the production of crisis demands close attention not just to the immediate drama but also to everything that went before.

Crisis Metrics

The premise of this book is that contamination of the blood supply produced a crisis—more specifically, a *political* crisis—in France but not in the United States. By "political crisis" we mean that mobilization was targeted at individual state officials and, more broadly, at the policies, practices, and institutions of the state that appeared (as Grémy clearly believed) to "endanger society at large." The French state was, at one and the same time, targeted, endangered, and held responsible for reform.

There are several metrics—none wholly satisfactory in themselves, somewhat more persuasive when taken together—by which to gauge empirically the degree to which an occurrence rises to the level of political crisis. Alexander suggests that key actors in the production of political crisis are journalists and lawyers "upon whose successful performances the actual unfolding of societalization [breaching boundaries between the private and the public sphere] depends" (Alexander 2018:1049). Performance of journalists may be measured by numbers of pertinent articles published; performance of lawyers by the numbers of court cases brought and of indictments and convictions. (Lawyers—and even journalists—are adept at keeping things *out* of the public sphere should the occasion require.) Other less quantifiable measures include statements and actions by political figures contemporaneous with the events in question and retrospective evaluations by historians.

Newspaper Articles

In Figure 1.1 we compare the publication trajectories (1985–1995) of articles containing the key words AIDS and BLOOD between newspapers with a national circulation in each country, *Le Monde* (France) and the *New York Times* (United States). Attention to the blood/AIDS nexus had trailed off in both countries between 1985 and 1990 and, although differently inflected, in neither case was media attention before 1990 focused on contaminated blood as a public scandal. The marked *Le Monde* spike in 1991–1993 reflects the media storm precipitated by Casteret's article.

Litigation

Writing in 1999, Bayer estimated that in the United States "300–500" cases had been filed by persons infected by the blood supply; defendants were blood product manufacturers, blood banks, hospitals, and physicians

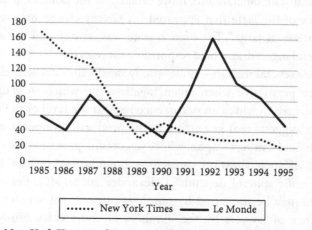

Figure 1.1 *New York Times* and *Le Monde*, "Blood" and "AIDS" Coverage ("*sang*" et "*sida*").

(1999:37).[16] In the same publication, Steffen gave the number of cases filed in France as "nearly 2000" (1999:116). Based on estimates of the number of AIDS cases among hemophiliacs and individuals infected through transfusion, these figures indicate that close to 100% of persons who acquired AIDS through the blood supply filed suit in France, as compared to between 3% and 5% in the United States. *In none of the U.S. cases were government officials among the defendants.* In France, by contrast, not only were high-level officials investigated and brought to trial, but the French Constitution was amended to ensure that ministers of state might be indicted as well (Steffen 1999, Chauveau 2011). In the course of litigation that ended only in 2003, a former prime minister, a former health minister, and a former minister of social affairs were formally placed "under investigation" by the courts along with twenty-one additional blood sector officials, ministerial aids, and senior civil servants.

Contemporaneous Statements

On November 3, 1991, Georgina Dufoix, French health minister during the critical period of the mid-1980s, responding to public furor over Casteret's revelations seven months earlier of blood supply contamination and massive infection of hemophiliacs, stated on national television that she was "responsible but not guilty," eliciting further furor and calls by the opposition party for charges to be brought "at the highest political level" (Nau and Nouchi 1991d. *Le Monde*, November 5). A week later, François Mitterrand, president of the French Republic, said in a televised speech that "we need a law, we need Parliament as a whole to be involved in the measures that have to be taken to compensate [for] damages which can never be entirely compensated" (cited in Steffen 1999:113). One month later, Parliament unanimously approved legislation establishing a public compensation plan.

The first U.S. congressional hearing on the safety of the blood supply in July 1990, went largely unnoticed by the American media.[17] Neither this

---

[16] In 1994 the judge certifying a class action suit on behalf of infected hemophiliacs noted that 300 cases were pending nationwide. This seems consistent with Bayer's figure five years later. Nevertheless, since defendants (blood banks, blood products manufacturers) were successful in quashing many of these suits before they came to trial, the exact number is difficult to estimate.

[17] More precisely, we retrieved five articles that covered this hearing at the time it occurred. Two of these five were duplicate wire service stories. Only one paper, the *Philadelphia Inquirer* (an excellent but wholly regional newspaper with a strong history of interest in the blood story), put the hearing on the front page.

hearing nor the hearings on the bill that established the Ryan White Care Act, occurring at about the same time, are mentioned in major secondary sources on the blood affair in the United States (IOM 1995, Bayer 1999, Siplon 2002). Ryan White was a highly sympathetic young hemophiliac who died of AIDS; as an "innocent" and "deserving" victim, he provided essential political cover for Congress to pass a bill that authorized massive funding for healthcare to a population consisting predominantly of highly stigmatized gay men (Donovan 1996). *How* Ryan White became infected was essentially ignored. The "politics of restitution" central to the French case did not surface in the United States until much later, in the mid-1990s. When members of the Institute of Medicine (IOM) committee appointed to investigate the blood affair wanted to raise the issue of compensation, they were told by committee staff that "if their report broached the issue it would be excised in the review process" (Bayer 1999:45). On the question of compensation, the Clinton administration maintained "a studied silence" (Bayer 1999:48).

Judgments of History

Scholars' retrospective comments on the blood affair in France and the United States tell very different stories. French historian, François Cusset described the "tainted blood affair" in France as "the most serious political-medical tragedy of the post-war period" (2006:181); Paul Jankowski, professor of French history at Brandeis, called it "the most resounding political scandal of the late twentieth century" (2008:166). French political scientist Monica Steffen, remarking on the legal drama, observed, "it was the trial [of senior officials] that would rivet the attention of the French public and that would mark the experience of France as unique among other nations that confronted the iatrogenic tragedy of AIDS and blood" (1999:117). Marmor, Dillon, and Scher, after reviewing detailed accounts of eight countries' experience with this tragedy, including France and the United States, stated flatly of the United States, "there was no crisis, either governmental or non-governmental" (1999:361).

Each of these elements—newspaper coverage, litigation, contemporary and retrospective statements—is consistent with our premise that political crisis was present in the French and absent in the American case. Among the often-cited rewards of research into disasters and crises is that "institutions reveal much about themselves when under stress or in crisis, when they face the unexpected as well as the routine" (Burawoy 1998:14). Our hypothesis in the present case is that revelations will come not only from crisis—the dog barked—but also from careful examination of why in comparable circumstances the dog remained silent.

Others have raised the question of France's "unique" response (in addition to Steffen cited above, see also Feldman 2000 and Chauveau 2011), but less attention has been paid to explaining the absence of crisis in the United States, perhaps because—as observed by Fligstein and McAdam—absence of crisis is predictable, "destabilization is rare" (2012:20). Among the few observers to question this "absence" (and the first chronologically, to our knowledge) was the author (*rapporteur*) for the French National Assembly's report on the blood affair in France. Based on the inquiries of his commission, "underestimation of the risk was universal . . . all countries comparable to France experienced, at about the same time, the same debates and the same difficulties." Yet, "ours is the only country where the drama of the years 1984–85 was politicized" (AN 1993:210). The rapporteur was particularly struck by the "solidarity" of officials in the United States in support of its government "irrespective of their own political position" but observed that accounting for this difference was beyond the scope of the commission's responsibilities. Our mission is not only to account for France's uniqueness but also the relative *sang-froid* (so to speak) of the United States to which the rapporteur could only—somewhat ruefully—allude. As the Tillys observed about collective action in nineteenth-century Europe, "an explanation of protest, rebellion, or collective violence that cannot account for its absence is no explanation at all" (Tilly et al. 1975:12).

Sober chroniclers of crises past warn us to beware of the "retrospective fallacy": "retrospection corrects history, altering the past to make it consistent with the present, implying that errors should have been anticipated" (Vaughan 1996:393, see also IOM 1995:2). Vaughan contrasts this "politics of blame" unfavorably with "systematic research" that reveals "the meanings of actions to insiders at the time." (Vaughan 1996:393). Nevertheless, "causal stories" that identify victims and perpetrators and assign blame are the stuff of politics as one side "seeks to push a problem into the realm of human purpose [blame], the other side seeks to push it away from intent back toward the realm of nature" (Stone 1988:158). Although we will necessarily have much to say about the choices made by blood bankers, political figures, public health officials, and other actors in the HIV/blood drama, grounded in their institutional locations and in the meanings of their actions at the time, our aim in this book is not to explain a public health disaster but to account for the transformation of that disaster into a political crisis. For the latter purpose, we must address "the politics of blame" in as much detail as we do the drama itself.

American Exceptionalism

The blood story in the United States not only departs markedly from the blood story in France but also from the country's history of managing risks and regulating dangerous products. Prasad began her history of failed efforts to fight poverty in America, *The Land of Too Much*, with a narrative of the Food and Drug Administration's (FDA) Frances Kelsey protecting the American public from thalidomide. Prasad's intent was to counter the misreading of the United States as a weak noninterventionist state in comparison with the supposedly interventionist Europeans who embraced thalidomide. "The most surprising fact about [the thalidomide case was that] it was the laissez-faire United States—the country that supposedly hates state intervention, the country allegedly most favorable to the market—that was the most successful at using the state to protect consumers from a pharmaceutical company wanting to market a dangerous drug, while the drug was welcomed all over statist Europe" (Prasad 2012:6). The rise of toxic tort litigation in the United States centered on a debate "about how to strike an equitable and efficient balance between the producers and the innocent victims of toxic chemicals" tells a similar story (Jasanoff 1995:118). Given this history, the reluctance of the American state to protect the "innocent victims" of the "dangerous drug" that was human blood is surely counterintuitive: "Blood banking enjoys protection unique to any other product or industry in the world" (executive director of the American Association of Blood Banks, cited in Eckert 1992:251). Equally counterintuitive—indeed inexplicable—is the fact that this paradox has received so little notice. Among the FDA's "vast [and] remarkable powers" (Carpenter 2010:1) is responsibility for regulation of the American blood supply domestically, as well as overseas insofar as blood enters the domestic supply chain. Yet the blood story is entirely absent from Carpenter's magisterial work on the FDA. Hilts devotes a few lines to what he describes as the FDA's "victory" in 1992 over delinquent Red Cross blood banks (2003:291); Richert's (2014) account of the FDA in the Reagan era, when HIV contamination of the blood supply occurred (and despite his subtitle, "Prescription for Scandal"), makes no reference to the regulatory failure reflected in HIV contamination of the blood supply.

Methods

This is a case-comparative study of parallel and contrasting events as they played out in two countries over the same time period. Although there are critical differences in history and in political culture and structure between France and the United States—and these differences are key elements in our story—the two countries during the period of investigation were *broadly similar* as industrialized democracies with advanced scientific and medical establishments and *similar more specifically* in many details of the blood contamination story. Our choice of the United States to compare with France was driven not only by the stark contrast in response to the event of HIV/blood contamination, but also by our ability to hold constant at least some of the many potential sources of variation that might explain this contrast (see, e.g., Ragin and Becker 1992).

The data we analyze in this investigation are multiple texts: interviews, archives, newspaper articles, official reports, parliamentary and congressional hearings, memoirs, and legal documents (sources are listed in Appendix C "Original Sources"). We call particular attention to two unique sources. First, we were able to access French health ministry cabinet archives not normally available to scholars for periods central to our story, 1988–1990 and 1992–1993. Second, our sources include multiple oral history interviews with key players both in France and in the United States.[18] We approach these texts not primarily as "information" (although, while we approach it critically, we do not ignore the information these texts convey) but as narratives or stories that attempt to "make sense" of conflicting and contested streams of information. Our approach to this analysis is informed by the work of social movement scholars on "framing processes" (Snow et al. 1986, Benford and Snow 2000, Swidler 1986); by Deborah Stone's (1988) deconstruction of "causal stories"; by recent work on "sensemaking" by Weick 1995, Abolafia 2020, and others; and by studies of "organizational discourse" analysis (e.g., Gabriel 2004). Benford and Snow observe that "movement actors are

---

[18] Including archived oral histories (fifteen) and interviews conducted in person by the authors (fourteen), the totals for each country are France (thirteen), United States (fifteen).

viewed as *signifying agents* actively engaged in the production and maintenance of meaning for constituents, antagonists, and bystanders or observers"
(2000:613, emphasis added). Not only movement actors but also political
and institutional actors more broadly behave as "signifying agents" engaged
in the social production of meaning for rhetorical and persuasive purposes
(Fligstein and McAdam 2012:47ff). When it comes to social problems,
as Stone points out, "we look for causes not only to understand how the
world works but to *assign responsibility*" (Stone 1988:147). How "causes" are
portrayed (accidental, inadvertent, intentional) has a great deal to do with
attributions of responsibility.

How did the multiple actors in the HIV/blood contamination story
(journalists, blood bankers, officials, hemophiliacs, lawyers) "make sense"
of its various elements? The analytic steps we followed to answer this question were (1) identification of principal actors in the policy and political
drama surrounding HIV infection of the blood supply and of their relations of cooperation and power; (2) creation of timelines of critical events
across multiple domains (e.g., health, administrative, political, civil society
institutions) within the larger narrative; (3) discovery of meaning (knowledge and problem framing, attributions of responsibility for causing and
coping with the problem); (4) elucidation of underlying political processes
of struggle over ownership and domination of the terrain represented by the
cross-cutting fields of HIV and the blood supply.

As we have earlier observed, there is a large French literature on the "*affaire du sang*." We emphasize that our narrative does not change the existing empirical story so much as add substantial depth through our access
to French government archives; interviews with key players, including cabinet officials; and key documents and reports. Second, because our analytic
strategy requires that we tell an empirical story in the first part of the book
and then interpret and theorize that story in the second part, there is a certain amount of inevitable repetition between the two halves. We have tried to
keep repetition to a minimum but, regrettably, we have not been able to avoid
it altogether.

Plan of the Book

This first chapter poses the central questions this book project was designed
to answer. It is intended to set the stage historically and theoretically for

what will follow. Chapter 2 describes the history and organization of blood services in France and the United States after the Second World War when blood was transformed from an artisanal to a mass-produced commodity. Chapter 2 provides essential background for the series of narratives that are the data on which comparative analysis to unravel the social production of crisis are based. The next three chapters under the broad label "Blood Stories" are crisis narratives. They tell the stories of HIV contamination of the blood supply, how it became a full-blown political crisis in France (and not in the United States), and the social mobilization of the contaminated (principally hemophiliacs but in France transfusees as well). The first two of these three chapters, titled "Act 1—Before the Storm, 1981–1985" (Chapter 3) and "Act 2—The Storm Breaks, 1986–1995" (Chapter 4) are fairly straightforward chronological accounts of the unfolding blood story in each of the two countries. Chapter 5 overlaps Chapter 4 in time and describes the gradual mobilization of hemophiliacs as political communities organized to assert their interests and demand recognition and compensation from courts and from the state. Chapters 6 through 8 we have labeled "Blood Epistemology." "Epistemology" is defined as study of the nature and grounds of knowledge especially with reference to its limits and validity. These chapters examine and compare how various parties (courts, official commissions, political bodies, the press, academics) in the two countries framed what was "known" about HIV in the blood supply, when it was known, the limits and validity of that knowledge, and who (if anyone) among the multiple actors in this drama was "responsible"—for knowing, and for acting on that knowledge.

In Chapter 9, "The Social Production of Political Crisis," we will draw on our empirical data to more fully develop our conceptual framework to explain the social production of political crisis. Although we believe this framework has wide application (and bears some resemblance to existing crisis frameworks (see, e.g., Fligstein and McAdam 2012:20, Alexander 2018, 2019), we arrived at it only after long immersion in the details of our particular case. The final chapter (Chapter 10, "Conclusion: Crisis and Change") is a series of reflections, first, on the ongoing ripples from the blood scandal in France; second, on the reach of our conceptual framework; and, third, on the contingent politics of epidemics, drawing on and extending the work of Charles Rosenberg (1989). Both Sewell (1992, 1996) in his theorizing of "events" and Fligstein and McAdam (2012) in their "theory of fields" define crises in part by their consequences. Among the consequences of the French blood crisis were profound changes in the meaning and institutions of public health, in legal norms about victim compensation, and in the precautionary principle. Second, we extend the reach of our conceptual framework, comparing two events in American public health history with very different "crisis" outcomes. Finally, we examine our case for what it can tell us about the politics of epidemic disease. That there is a "politics" of epidemic disease should come as no surprise to anyone who has lived through the era of COVID-19. We are struck as much by the early parallels between France and the United States in patterns of response to the misunderstood and uncertain threat of AIDS in the blood supply as by their later divergence, raising questions about the role not only of disease characteristics but also of history, culture, politics, institutions, and period in conditioning countries' highly contingent responses to epidemic challenge. In reflecting on these questions, we draw heavily on Charles Rosenberg's seminal essay on the AIDS epidemic, "What is an Epidemic?" (1989).

2
The Social Life of Blood, 1948–1980

Both France and the United States struggled in the decades immediately following the Second World War to find consensus on the meaning of blood. Consensus was reached with relative ease in France and only with great difficulty in the United States. Struggles over meaning and over the organization of blood services were inseparably linked and mutually constitutive. The nature of these struggles and their different resolutions are key to understanding why a blood crisis erupted in France in the 1980s and why there was no such crisis in the United States.

World War II was the crucible in which the infinite possibilities of blood as a therapeutic technology were forged and made visible to the world. Before the war, transfusion of whole blood was an artisanal process—arm to arm, donor and recipient lying side by side connected by a Y-shaped tube—resorted to primarily in emergencies.[1] Donors were on call and were paid for their time without moral compunction.[2] Blood and blood transfusion were of interest to a small group of medical and scientific specialists. By the end of the war, the blood field was transformed by rapid advances in technology, by new models of blood collection, and by the wholesale entry of U.S.-based pharmaceutical companies into the business of blood.

World War II drove advances in blood technology on two fronts. First, in the preservation and transport of whole blood, obviating the necessity for donor and recipient to meet. Second, in the fractionation of blood into its cellular components, each with its own distinct and valuable therapeutic properties: first chronologically, the separation of blood plasma— the liquid that carries those components (and can itself be transfused

---

[1] Hermitte points to ties of affection between hemophiliacs in this period before the Second World War and "their" donor with whom they had frequent occasion to meet on account of recurrent hemorrhages (1996:98). Starr characterizes arm-to-arm donation as "blood on the hoof" (2002:53).

[2] Professional blood donation was funded in Paris as a high society charity (Chauveau 2007:36); elite physicians in New York City organized the Blood Betterment Association, recruiting carefully selected professional donors committed to "good health and discipline" (Starr 2002:60).

The Social Production of Crisis. Constance A. Nathanson and Henri Bergeron, Oxford University Press.
© Oxford University Press 2023. DOI: 10.1093/oso/9780197682487.003.0002

directly)—from red blood cells and, later, the breakdown of plasma into separate proteins including, among others, the factors that promote blood coagulation. Hemophilia is a sex-linked hereditary bleeding disorder caused by a deficiency in the body's ability to synthesize proteins necessary for blood clotting. Females are carriers, but the condition is expressed almost entirely in males. Prior to the isolation of the anti-hemophilia factor (AHF) and its preparation in concentrated form, hemophiliacs depended on transfusions to manage severe and crippling hemorrhages, often requiring extended hospitalization. Technological advances in the 1960s and 1970s led, first, to the development of freeze-dried plasma rich in AHF and, a few years later, to an even more highly concentrated version made by pooling thousands of units of plasma—from thousands of donors. These new technologies were greeted enthusiastically by hemophiliacs and their families; only haltingly and with reluctance would their downsides come to be recognized.

The massive demand for blood created by the war (amplified by the technologies we have described) in the United States led to organized blood donation campaigns on a large scale, carried out by the American Red Cross on behalf of the military. Blood donation in France was complicated by the German occupation: groups of paid donors tied to hospitals continued to donate under the Vichy government; a second stream of voluntary donations was organized by the French resistance and served both its members and the allied armies after D-day.

U.S. military requirements led to the development and production of blood products (primarily for the treatment of shock from blood loss) on a scale far beyond anything undertaken before the war. "Within the first half of America's entry into the war, a chain of manufacturing had been developed to produce dried plasma on a national scale" (Starr 2002:110). Multiple universities and nine pharmaceutical companies were under contract to the American government; "this degree of cooperation between universities and industry was unprecedented" (Starr 2002:111). By the end of the war, a new pharmaceutical-manufacturing industry had been created in the United States, and its raw material was blood. There were no opportunities during the war for comparable industrial development in France, and—as we shall see—what opportunities there were after the war were quickly shut down. Nevertheless, blood had, in both countries, become an invaluable national resource.

Constructing and Deconstructing Blood: France

"The human body—and its parts—has long been a target for commodification within myriad cultural settings" (Sharp 2000:287); among the earliest (and perhaps least contested) targets has been human blood. The meanings of blood in France encompassed not only its moral status as a bodily fluid but also the moral status of its components (blood products), the act of blood donation, the donor, and the blood system within which each of these elements circulated. Before the upheaval of 1991–1992, these elements were inseparable both in French law and in popular understanding. Their interconnection was forcefully articulated in a 1958 opinion by the Conseil d'État:

> Dignity requires that the human body should not become an object of commerce, neither as a whole nor in its elements. And it is not sufficient to decide that this commerce must exclude all profit; there must also be assurance of a sharp distinction between operations on human blood and its products and all commercial activity. . . . As for solidarity, that is only possible when those who give blood know that it and its derivatives will not, directly or indirectly become the objects of commerce. . . . Blood donation is a form of active solidarity. . . . Between an honorable sacrifice and degrading traffic, there is a single difference: total disinterestedness. (Conseil d'État, 9 mai 1958, cited in Hermitte 1996:134)

Blood—in this reading—was intrinsic to personal integrity and human dignity, its commercialization no less abhorrent than human slavery; *blood donation*—in the form of a gift, and only as a gift—was both an expression of reciprocal social ties and critical to their construction; social ties created by blood donation were the building blocks of national solidarity.[3] Essential to the realization of these values insisted the author of the Conseil's opinion was that the entire system of "operations on human blood" be not for profit—outside the economic market—and that these operations encompass not only whole blood but also blood products. The economic model reflected in this opinion incorporates much the same ideological critique of market

---

[3] Drawing on another example from the arena of public health, France was initially unfriendly to antismoking propaganda in part because smoking—like blood donation—was seen as a form of solidarity, the creation of social ties over a friendly cigarette (Nathanson 2007).

exchange later embraced by Richard Titmuss, centering on the destructive social, moral, and cultural effects of the commodification of blood (and of commodification more generally) (Titmuss [1970] 1997, Zelizer 1988).

This opinion upheld a law passed by the French Parliament on July 21, 1952, titled, "Utilisation thérapeutique de produits d'origine humaine" (therapeutic use of products of human origin). The 1952 law created a framework for the organization of blood transfusion in France that lasted essentially unchanged for forty years, until the beginning of the 1990s (Chauveau 2007:23). It (along with regulatory statutes issued in 1954) codified rules for blood transfusion that had been issued in a somewhat ad hoc fashion by the Ministry of Health dating back to French liberation from the German occupation in 1944. Behind this law lay a complex history of sometimes competing and sometimes converging interests and ideologies against a background of inexorable advance in blood technology and ever-increasing demand for the "raw material" that powered that advance, human blood.

France ended the war with a chaotic mix of public (hospital) and private entities engaged in the collection, processing, and transfusion of blood, organized under different (largely private) administrative auspices and with different organizational forms.[4] Hospitals that had been collecting and transfusing blood before and during the war continued to do so; the French military had its own blood system, first in Algeria and later on the mainland. The most consequential of these entities, however, was the clandestine system developed by the French resistance movement during the occupation. Committed to the ethical principal of voluntary—unpaid—donation, militants of the resistance moved quickly following the liberation to conquer new terrain and extend their influence through donor associations and publications.[5] "The spirit of solidarity tied to the war gave birth to a new model of the blood donor, the benevolent and voluntary donor as opposed to the paid donor" (Chauveau 2007:48). Through their publication, *Le Donneur de Sang*, militants of the *bénévolat* were aggressive in their attacks on paid donation and on the donors themselves, going so far as to accuse

---

[4] Our principal sources for the following account of the French blood system as it emerged after the Second World War are *Le Sang et le Droit* by Marie-Angèle Hermitte (1996) and the comprehensive, detailed, and insightful narrative presented by Sophie Chauveau as the first volume of her professorial thesis (Habilitation), "Du don au marché: Politiques du sang en France années 1940-années 2000" (2007) ("From Gift to Marketplace: Blood Politics in France from 1940 to 2000").

[5] *Le Donneur de Sang* was published from at least 1950. In 1958, the name was changed to *Le Donneur de Sang Bénévole*.

paid hospital donors who had continued this practice during the war of "collaboration" (i.e., with the Nazis).[6] These attacks—and the organized groups behind them—were effective not only because they were able to capitalize on the spirit of national solidarity created by the war but also because the French government depended on a privately funded system of voluntary donations to sustain the country's blood supply.

Wanting to bring some order and technical supervision to this chaos, as well as to ensure that the end of the war did not bring an end to blood donation, the Ministry of Health intervened in 1946 to create the Commission Consultative de Transfusion Sanguine (CCTS) (Blood Transfusion Commission) and in 1947 issued a series of regulations setting the minimum requirements for a blood center to be officially recognized (*agréé*) by the state.The requirements were, indeed, minimal but nonetheless of enormous significance: whatever their auspices, public or private, blood centers were designated a *public service*, nonprofit, and off limits to any commercial enterprise; to ensure "competent" management, center directors must be approved by the "highest authority in these matters," the CCTS. As Chauveau points out, the CCTS was from its earliest incarnation in 1946 composed of transfusion elites, the doctors in charge of major transfusion centers, at first in Paris and later in the provinces as well. Center directors were appointed from these same elite medical circles.

An additional and critical element of this structure was its character, in American legislative parlance, as an "unfunded mandate." Government intervention (including the fixing of prices for blood products) did not come with government funding or, indeed, more than minimal central direction. The office for blood services was part of a small bureau within the health administration, staffed by a single administrator with multiple other responsibilities.[7] The French government had neither the funds nor the personnel to create a national, centralized blood service. It was and continued for the next four decades to be dependent on the same local and regional initiatives that created blood centers immediately after the war. We will use the case of Lyon, described in some detail by Sophie Chauveau, to illustrate how this system came about.

---

[6] Hermitte points out that in this period voluntary donation was advocated entirely on the basis of principle with no reference to public health. It was only later, once the principle had been firmly established, that the higher *quality* of blood donated voluntarily was argued. Organized blood donors continued their attack on paid donation through 1976 when the final bastion of paid donation (for plasmapheresis) in France (the Institute Mérieux) was persuaded to stop remunerating its donors.

[7] This administrator was sometimes, but not invariably, a physician.

Lyon is the third-largest city in France after Paris and Marseilles, located in the central part of the country in the department of the Rhône. Chauveau describes the history of its postwar blood center as originating with a letter from the Conseil National de la Résistance (National Council of the Resistance) sent in 1944 to a professor of hematology in Lyon (Louis Revol) asking that a center be established in that city for processing blood and blood products. Revol proposed, and was instrumental in creating, a regional center that pulled together resources from the local university hospital's existing transfusion services, from army surplus equipment and supplies, and from the clandestine blood services organized under the German occupation. Revol's plan envisioned a center that would carry out *both* whole blood transfusion *and* the manufacture of blood products, relying on voluntary donors and family members (professional donors would be "too expensive"). It would have the status of an autonomous nonprofit organization and would be financed by the hospital, by the army (this was 1944), by the sale of blood products, and by charitable contributions. Chauveau suggests that Revol's plan served as a template for subsequent ministerial orders regarding the organization of blood centers in France.

The Lyon regional blood center was formally established in October 1945. The composition of its various administrative committees, consisting of prominent physicians and local political elites, was characteristic of actors in the blood field in France at the time.[8] The original Board of Directors, for example, included representatives from the departmental public health authority (Direction Départementale des Affaires Sanitaires et Sociales [DDASS]), the local hospital association and its medical committee, the army medical services, the Red Cross, the health insurance system (l'Union générale des caisses d'Assurances Sociales), and the local donor association (la Mutuelle du Sang).[9] Other local authorities were added later, and a patron committee was set up to solicit charitable donations. Revol was charged with the center's medical direction, a post he occupied for the next thirty years.[10]

---

[8] The first community blood banks in the United States were quite similar in their reliance on local medical, social, and political elites for administrative, fundraising, and other forms of support.

[9] There was considerable overlap in the characteristics of the Lyon CTS Board of Directors and those of its counterpart in Kansas City in about the same period as described in testimony before the FTC (*In the Matter of Community Blood Bank of* Kansas City 1966). The main difference was the presence on the Lyon board of local public health and insurance authorities and of blood *donors*.

[10] Revol's tenure in office was the norm rather than the exception; once appointed, local blood services directors retained their positions more or less indefinitely (Chauveau 2007:93).

The Lyon case was unusual in only one respect: its organization as a nonprofit blood center that encompassed all phases of the blood industry from collection to the manufacture of blood products came about in direct opposition—led by the local medical establishment—to an alternative model that would have mimicked the American system of separating the noncommercial collection and processing of whole blood from the commercial—and highly profitable—business of blood products. Charles Mérieux, an enterprising lyonnaise physician, returned from a French government sponsored trip to the United States immediately after the war full of enthusiasm about American blood technology and eager to transplant it to Lyon. His medical colleagues would have none of that: "in giving in to the demands of Doctor Mérieux, we would be transferring our blood center over to [Mérieux's organization]," and the center, organized in the national interest, would end up in the unacceptable position of benefiting a private enterprise.[11] Mérieux was not alone, however, in his advocacy for a dual system. Parliamentary hearings on the 1952 law revealed a vocal minority who wanted to completely separate the status of blood at the point of collection from blood products, which should be subject to the rules of the market. Their voices were overwhelmed by the majority—supported by the official parliamentary reporter on the law and by powerful donor associations with their strong ties to politicians at the local level—who favored a completely voluntary and nonprofit system, a "harbor in the heart of the market economy" (Chauveau 2007:126). Interestingly, the law itself made no reference to blood products as distinct from whole blood, nor did it expressly prohibit paid donation.[12]

The *principle* of state responsibility for the medical care of its citizens was accepted by French political authorities in the aftermath of World War I. Its implementation and the expansion of national health insurance to increasing categories of the population occurred in fits and starts with a great leap forward under the resistance government immediately following the end of

[11] Chauveau suggests that there was considerable rivalry between Revol and Mérieux both of whom had played important roles in the Second World War (in the army and the resistance, respectively) and thought of themselves as entitled to lead Lyon's new blood center. We owe detailed information on the development of the Lyon blood center to Doctor Mérieux's extensive notes. The "Institut Mérieux," founded in 1897, continues in existence as a family-owned and -controlled pharmaceutical company based in Lyon. Our point is that local doctors' opposition to the Mérieux model very likely had more complex origins than opposition to private enterprise alone.

[12] Blood centers were occasionally forced to accept paid donation in cases of emergency (as were community blood banks in the United States).

World War II. The influence of local physicians—long-standing chiefs of hospital services, as in the case of Dr. Revol, who not infrequently held the offices of both mayor and member of Parliament—on the organization of healthcare services was, nonetheless, profound, no more so than in the case of blood services.

Within this context, the French blood system was shaped by an ideological commitment—powered initially by the resistance movement and sustained by large and nationally organized donor associations—to a voluntary, non-profit system; by an ever-increasing demand for blood and blood products; by the inability and/or unwillingness of the French government to fund and staff a centrally managed blood service; and by the resulting concentration of power in the hands of donor associations and medical elites at the local and regional level. "It is a system with extraordinary power in French political life. The blood donor associations, the transfusions system, the elite transfusion doctors, this is no small thing. . . . It is a major power in the true sense of the word. It is very impressive, the biggest names in medicine are part of this system" (Evin cabinet official, interview by author, November 4, 2010). The serious administrative and financial dysfunctions of this system had been made clear in a series of official reports beginning in 1971 (see, e.g., Blin and Bestaux 1971).[13] But not until the blood crisis did the government have sufficient leverage to bring about its reform.

It is tempting, as Hermitte does (albeit with caution), to see this system, and the AIDS disaster it invited, as driven almost entirely by blind faith in the moral virtue of a non-market system and, by extension, in the purity of its donors and, ipso facto, of its output in blood and blood products. This is a case, however, in which ideological, political, and economic interests converged. Faced with increasing demand, the central government had neither the resources nor the capacity to organize blood collection on the necessary scale, to set up blood centers at the local level, or to engage in the industrial production of blood products (fractionation). These constraints created a highly unbalanced field of power in which donor associations and the high priests of medicine at the local level—fractionators in particular—held almost all the cards, and the government officially in charge held very few.

---

[13] Blin and Bestaux were highly placed civil servants in, respectively, the French Treasury and the Finance Ministry. The frustration of these investigators in the face of the chaotic administration of blood services was palpable in their report. They were clearly horrified.

Constructing and Deconstructing Blood: United States

Americans also gave blood with patriotic fervor during World War II , responding to blood drives on behalf of the military managed by the American National Red Cross (ARC) at the instance of the federal government. For civilians, there were hospital blood banks, similar to those in France. With the end of the war, however, the differences between the two countries became stark, even startling in the rapidity with which these differences emerged and in their profound implications for how the blood supply would be understood and managed in the United States. The parameters of blood collection, processing, and transfusion of whole blood and the manufacture of blood products were no less ideologically driven—and, indeed, politicized—in the United States than in France, and questions about the role of the market and of "voluntary" versus "paid" blood were equally central. But the answers to those questions were very different. In both countries ideological and organizational conflicts played out largely within the blood system itself, despite the nominally greater engagement of the state in France. The American federal government took little interest in the blood system until the early 1970s.

Meanings of blood and modes of organization for its supply were inseparable and, in the United States, consisted of multiple ideologically irreconcilable and mutually competitive systems: until the early 1970s the supply of whole blood was split among hospital and small independent blood banks; the much larger, loosely coordinated banks run by the ARC; and commercial for-profit blood centers.[14] Blood products were supplied by five fully commercial pharmaceutical enterprises. Donor organizations, so prominent in shaping the French blood system, were (and are) nonexistent in the United States.[15]

---

[14] The relative importance of each source of blood varied widely across the country. Douglas Starr asserts that "for-profit blood centers never constituted more than a fifth of the nation's collection capacity" (1998:189); the remainder was close to evenly split between the Red Cross and independent voluntary blood banks. However, in New York City in the late 1950s and early 1960s almost half the supply came from commercial banks.

[15] Donors to Red Cross banks were recruited from businesses and unions, not from groups organized in their capacity as blood donors. For example, "Within the first year [of opening a Red Cross blood bank in Rochester, NY] the Eastman Kodak Company signed on as a donor group, and with its large and willing population provided an assured donor base" (Kennedy 235). Insofar as there was "donor" representation in the United States, it was in the hands of those who extracted the raw material, not in those who supplied it.

The first steps toward a postwar blood system in this country coincided with the high point of "socialized medicine" as a battle cry in the Cold War. For two decades beginning in the late 1940s the American Medical Association (AMA), local medical societies, and their political allies mounted national lobbying campaigns ("the most expensive lobbying effort in American history"; Starr 1982:285) and went to court against the threat of "socialized medicine" as represented by a proposal for national health insurance espoused by the Truman administration and by prepaid group or cooperative health plans that sprang up around the country in the 1950s and 1960s. When in 1947 the ARC authorized its local chapters to establish blood banks grounded in ethical principles similar to those in France, it came almost immediately under attack from organized medicine. ARC's principles—blood was a community responsibility and should be donated voluntarily and supplied without charge to anyone in need—were quickly labeled as socialized medicine.[16] Within six months local physician-dominated (largely hospital) blood banks had formed a competing national organization, the American Association of Blood Banks (AABB), grounded in market-based principles that transfused blood should either be replaced (by family and friends) or paid for.[17] AABB had no objection to the Red Cross recruiting volunteers (although it initially took no position against paid donors); it objected powerfully to the ideas of "community responsibility" and "free" blood. And so, from its very beginnings, the American blood system was split into opposing ideological camps revolving around the contested relationship of money and blood and, inevitably, around the organizational and financial arrangements this relationship implied.[18]

Nowhere are the contrasting ideological perspectives of the French and the Americans more clearly revealed than in the contest between the U.S. Federal Trade Commission (FTC) and the Community Blood Bank of Kansas City, a legal drama that played out in Congress, in FTC hearing rooms, and in the courts in the 1950s and 1960s. Most striking was the position taken by the FTC, among the oldest independent regulatory agencies in the United

[16] Given its role during the Second World War, ARC's opponents also saw it as a quasi-government organization, adding fuel to the cry of "socialized medicine!"

[17] Under the perceived threat of national health insurance in 1934, the AMA had enunciated its own principle that "the immediate cost [of medical service] should be borne by the patient if able to pay at the time the service is rendered," a principle it continued to defend in multiple venues through the rest of the twentieth century (Starr 2002:300).

[18] Over time, as blood morphed into a highly diverse collection of products and demand increased, the ARC itself became a multimillion-dollar industry.

States, that blood was a commodity and subject to all the laws of trade and commerce. In May 1955 doctors and hospital administrators of Kansas City were informed by letter that a new "commercial" blood bank had opened its doors in their city. As described in detail by the FTC hearing examiner, this development was met with considerable hostility by the local medical establishment. The question before the FTC was whether this hostility— taking the form of refusal to procure blood from a bank that operated "for profit"—amounted to a conspiracy in restraint of trade. The FTC concluded that it did and stated its reasons with exemplary clarity: first, "whole blood (human) is viable human tissue mixed with an anticoagulant in a sterile container which must be stored and refrigerated and *the admixture is a commodity and/or an article of commerce*"; second, "respondent corporations are engaged in 'trade' or 'business' for profit as those terms may properly be construed in the context of this case" (*In the Matter of Community Blood Bank* 1966:154).[19] Appearing in 1964 on behalf of a U.S. Senate bill that would have immunized blood banks from the FTC, a witness for the AMA made a surprisingly similar argument: "Human blood consists of living human tissue. It is a unique substance. It cannot be manufactured artificially, but must be obtained from another human being and, *of itself, has no intrinsic value*" (U.S. Senate 1964:86, emphasis added). From this (American) perspective, human blood was worthless without the technology that made it available for transfusion. The French position was diametrically opposed: blood had intrinsic value, and the question was whether that value—the human dignity it represented—was compromised by technological intervention. The answer by the Conseil d'État in 1958 was "no"—as long as collection was voluntary and profit did not intrude at any stage of the operation from collection to transfusion: "Between an honorable sacrifice and degrading traffic, there is a single difference: total disinterestedness" (Conseil d'État, 9 mai 1958, cited in Hermitte 1996:134).

Although the FTC examiner claimed not to doubt the sincerity of the physicians from Kansas City when they claimed to be guided by the "immorality" of trafficking in blood, his characterization of their behavior as "commerce" is unambiguous: "There has been and there now is a constant current and course of trade and commerce in blood between respondent Community

---

[19] The FTC hearing went on for most of the summer of 1963. "Almost one hundred witnesses were called and testified and almost one thousand exhibits were offered comprising about ten thousand pages of exhibits and over eight thousand pages of transcript. Over 800 pages of briefs and proposed findings were submitted" (*In the Matter of Community Blood Bank* 1966:21–22).

and other blood banks and hospitals" (*In the Matter of Community Blood Bank* 1966:737). Given these premises, Kansas City's doctors, hospitals, and blood banks were subject to the jurisdiction of the FTC and must "cease and desist" their illegal boycott of the commercial blood bank. The FTC's decision was overturned on appeal on the grounds that "nonprofit" hospitals and blood banks did not fall within the FTC's jurisdiction; the appellate court did not address the question of whether blood was a "commodity."

Aside from arguments about the moral status of blood, two issues were of grave concern to transfusion doctors and account for the attention paid to the Kansas City case. First, as Douglas Starr points out, "If blood became a product—like soda pop, for example—then other product-related statutes would kick in," including the Uniform Product Code, "a federal regulation adopted by all the states mandating that anything sold as an article of commerce carries an implied warranty" (1998:193). In other words, doctors, hospitals, and blood banks (not to speak of pharmaceutical companies) could be held strictly liable for injuries occasioned by transfusion or the use of blood products.[20] When the director of a large blood bank in Arizona told the United States Senate in 1964 that "one of the tragic aspects of the Kansas City decision in terms of its potential legal effect upon blood banks is the characterizing of blood as a commodity" (U.S. Senate 1964:77), he was not thinking about morality, but about potential liability.[21] "The doctrine of strict liability holds manufacturers accountable for injuries that are incurred from products that are inherently dangerous because diligence cannot fully eliminate their risks" (IOM 1995:223). The second cause for alarm was that the FTC's ruling threatened to expose all blood banks—not just the Kansas City bank—to the accusation of acting in restraint of trade: "The implications of this case are far-reaching and could have a profound effect on your operations, as well as those of every nonprofit community-serving blood bank in the United States" wrote the president of the Kansas City Community Blood Bank in an open letter to his colleagues soliciting funds to support the Community's legal battle against the FTC (Goldman 1964:207).[22] It is

[20] Ironically, given the powerful French aversion to treating blood as a consumer product, it was under just such a statute that in 1992 blood bankers were convicted in France.

[21] In direct response to the FTC's decision in the Kansas City case a bill was introduced in the U.S. Senate to exempt blood banks from antitrust laws.

[22] Organized medicine was no stranger to antitrust law. In 1943 the Supreme Court upheld the conviction of the AMA on antitrust violations for its actions against the Group Health Association of Washington, D.C. (Starr 1982:305). It seems likely that the hearing examiner's perspective on the actions of doctors in Kansas City was informed by this history; indeed, he specifically mentions the Group Health Association case as precedent.

no wonder that "news of the [FTC] decision triggered an outcry throughout the blood banking community" (Starr 2002:195). The FTC's ruling against Community was overturned, but the 1964 Senate bill went nowhere.

By far the most consequential outcome of these legal, administrative, and legislative battles were what are known as "blood shield" laws. The thrust of these laws, passed by almost every state in the two decades between 1955 and 1975, was to immunize blood banks and hospitals against legal liability for breach of warranty and/or from strict liability (liability without fault) in cases of patient injury from a "toxic blood" transfusion (principally—in that period—hepatitis).[23] Passage of these laws was precipitated by a line of court cases brought by patients who contracted hepatitis from blood transfusion, beginning with Gussie Perlmutter in 1954 (*Perlmutter v. Beth David Hospital* 1954). Perlmutter's lawyers argued that the transaction between the hospital and their client was a "sale" and therefore subject to implied warranties of merchantability and fitness for a particular purpose.[24] The New York Court of Appeals rejected this assertion, holding that the supplying of blood by the hospital was a "service" inseparable from medical treatment and therefore exempt from warranty liability. Unlike the FTC, which was only incidentally concerned with the meaning of blood as a "commodity," this question was central to *Perlmutter* and its progeny. The answer to it hinged on the legal and financial liability of blood banks and transfusion doctors, and they were quick to respond. "The vote [in *Perlmutter*] was close, the result was severely criticized, and it was by no means obvious that it would be followed. Physicians, hospital associations and blood bank groups therefore began to press for legislation to ward off the threat of strict liability" (Franklin 1972:474–75). State legislatures accomplished this feat by adopting the *Perlmutter* court's reasoning (and extending it): blood banking, blood transfusion, and blood processing (eventually including fractionation) were all a "service" not a "sale" and consequently exempt from attack under theories of implied warranty and strict liability.

There is ample evidence of the role played by organized medicine in the passage of these laws. In a 1969 statement, the AABB wrote that along with the AMA it "actively support[s] legislation to exempt blood and blood

---

[23] We use the phrase "toxic blood" advisedly instead of the more familiar "bad blood" to emphasize both the similarity between blood and other equally dangerous products (drugs, chemicals) that are subject to strict liability and, at the same time, the dissimilarity in their legal status.

[24] It is worth repeating that this is the identical argument made (successfully) against blood bankers by a French court in 1992.

derivatives from implied warranties (guarantees) of merchantability and fitness" (Franklin:475, n. 205). Franklin describes the lobbying activities of the Illinois State Medical Society in seeking to overturn a 1971 court decision that characterized toxic blood as a commodity analogous to "poisonous mushrooms" (*Cunningham v. MacNeal Memorial Hospital* 1970). "Their publication, *On the Legislative Scene* (March 5, 1971) urged members to 'contact your representative to explain the impact of the bill" and "write to (Illinois State) Senators with whom they were acquainted . . . explaining the urgency of this legislation and the desirability of keeping it out of the (Illinois State) Senate Judiciary Committee, which is composed entirely of attorneys [presumed to have an interest in the bill given that it shut off a potentially lucrative market in lawsuits against hospitals and blood banks]" (Franklin 1972:475, n. 205). The AABB's legal counsel, reflecting on this combat from the distance of several years, observed "because some courts reversed [*Perlmutter*] and also because we're aware that judges can change their minds—and sometimes do with remarkable swiftness and for remarkable reasons—we went to the state legislatures throughout the country" (cited in Eckert 1992:252).

This combat was remarkably one-sided. The political power of the AMA was at its height, and there was no organized opposition to blood shield laws from potential consumers (or even from lawyers).[25] Most striking is not only the absence of direct consumer pushback but also of more than passing reference in contemporary legal commentary to these laws' impact on consumers—recipients of blood whose interests were essentially erased by the preclusion of recovery grounded in warranty and/or strict liability. Only the few judges who had rejected *Perlmutter* (and whose judgments terrified the AABB and the AMA) took those interests into account: "The consequences of injury from dangerous blood should not 'fall upon the individual consumer who is entirely without fault" ' (cited in Eckert 1992:251). Even more puzzling is that in this same period "strict liability (liability without fault) [was replacing] negligence as the primary basis for compensating persons injured by defective products" (Jasanoff 1995:27). As reflected in the judicial language cited above, there was at the time "evolving judicial interest in

---

[25] Writing in 1970, contemporaneously with the passage of blood shield laws, Freidson described the AMA as "a private, national organization that has firm, well-organized roots in the local community and that through those local roots, has the greatest single influence on the organization of medical care in the United States" (1970:27). See also "The American Medical Association: Power, Purpose, and Politics in Organized Medicine," *The Yale Law Journal* 63, no. 7 (May 1954):937–1022.

compensating victims" (Jasanoff 1995:28). So, while the legal landscape with reference to other toxic substances was moving in a direction favorable to consumers, the landscape for toxic blood moved in reverse. This anomaly was acknowledged by the executive director of the AABB: "Blood banking enjoys protection unique to any other product or industry in the world. As far as I know, there is no other product that is immune from strict liability" (cited in Eckert 1992:251).

The provisions for blood supply that emerged in the United States after the Second World War were not a "system" in any meaningful sense of the word. They were a patchwork of arrangements fragmented along multiple ideological, economic, organizational, geographical, and technological fault lines without any central coordination—or interest—at the federal level. "Americans had never established a national policy. They left blood collection to the marketplace" (Starr 2002:188). Under conditions of increasingly high demand—"hospitals guzzled blood as voraciously as cars of the era consumed gasoline"—the result was what Starr labeled a "blood boom," a disorganized free-for-all of blood entrepreneurs eager to fill the gap between supply and demand.

This chaotic state of affairs did not go unnoticed within the blood field and, later, by the federal government. Between 1955 and 1980—when the first omens of the HIV epidemic appeared—there were two essentially fruitless efforts to create direction and coordination at the national level: the first promoted by the AMA, the second pushed but not led by the Nixon administration. The first of these attempts was the Joint Blood Council, established in 1955 with the goal of reconciling the conflicting positions of the ARC and the AABB—community responsibility grounded in voluntary donation versus individual responsibility and a pluralistic system (voluntary and paid donation) in line with fee-for-service medicine. The Joint Blood Council was hijacked by the AABB, policy differences between the AABB and the ARC proved irreconcilable, and the Council was dissolved in 1962 (Kennedy 1978).

The second effort was triggered in the early days of the Nixon administration by a sudden spike in public attention to the quality of the blood supply precipitated by a set of converging events: Richard Titmuss's indictment of the American blood system in *The Gift Relationship*, published in 1970; accompanying media attention to the problem of hepatitis in the blood supply; and an "increasingly vocal" consumer movement.[26] In 1971,

---

[26] The work of Kennedy (1978) and Douglas Starr (2002) offer ample documentation of these events. Kennedy states that *The Gift Relationship* provoked "an enormous response" from the

an ambitious freshman congressman from California garnered substantial public attention with a bill to create a National Blood Bank Program within Department of Health, Education, and Welfare with a director appointed by the president (Schmidt 1977:158). Lukewarm to this project, Nixon in March of 1972 asked the DHEW to "recommend to him as soon as possible a plan for developing a safe and efficient nationwide blood collection and distribution system" (Kennedy 1978:121). As Schmidt—himself deeply involved in blood politics at the time—recounted in a contemporary narrative of these events, Nixon's proposal was deliberately couched as a "policy" not a "program": "The use of the word 'policy' was clearly intended to transmit the message that the federal government in a Republican administration that was committed to a 'pluralistic society' did not want to run an organization to collect and distribute blood" (Schmidt 1977:160).

The language of this "policy" did nevertheless include an implied threat: "If the private sector is unable to make satisfactory progress toward implementing these policies, a legislative and/or regulatory approach would have to be considered" (cited in Schmidt 1977:164). The threat's immediate effect was to goad the antagonistic elements in the blood complex into a transient effort at cooperation, led by the AMA and formalized in late 1974 as the American Blood Commission (ABC). The ABC had no enforcement powers and very little money. Transient cooperation rapidly descended into internal squabbling along familiar lines, between the ARC and the AABB, and went so far as to trigger a lawsuit on behalf of the blood products industry accusing DHEW of embarking on "an illegal policy of eliminating commercialism in blood banking" (Kennedy 1978:126).[27] By 1979—with AIDS on

blood-banking community, although she does not specify the nature of that response. Starr observes that Garrett Allen, a surgeon and blood bank official with a long-standing concern about hepatitis in the blood supply, mailed a copy of *The Gift Relationship* to Nixon's secretary of HEW, Eliot Richardson (1998:226). Curiously, a highly critical report by the National Academy of Sciences published in 1970, *Evaluation of the Utilization of Human Blood Resources in the United States*, appears to have been largely ignored. The report described in detail the dysfunctional competition among entities within the blood "complex" (the word "system" was explicitly rejected as inapplicable to the fragmented condition of blood services in the United States), spelled out the dangers of hepatitis, and called for a federal agency to provide direction and coordination.

[27] Just as the ARC's move into the blood field in 1945 triggered the formation of the oppositional organization, AABB, so the creation of the American Blood Commission (ABC) triggered the formation of the equally oppositional American Blood Resources Association (ABRA), an organization of commercial firms dedicated to the manufacture of blood products. The ARC was perceived by these trade organizations as an arm of the federal government, antagonistic to private interests. It took the threat of AIDS to their common interests as blood suppliers to bring these antagonistic and highly competitive entities—temporarily—together.

the immediate horizon—the ABC "lay in ruins" (Starr 2002:256). It was disbanded in 1985.

This protracted struggle was arguably the high point of central government interest in the blood supply. Insofar as the intended outcome was a "nationwide blood collection and distribution *system,*" its failure was predictable (and was, indeed, predicted). Absent sustained federal interest and investment of resources (akin to the Nixon administration's investment in the Environmental Protection Agency), the effort was doomed by intense internal competition among blood suppliers, their combined—and equally intense—aversion to any semblance of government control, and the lack of an organized consumer constituency for blood safety parallel (for example) to the constituencies for tobacco control and the environment that emerged in the same period. The sustained *disinterest* of the federal government in creating a federal agency for blood was patent, made clear in DHEW comments on establishment of the ABC in 1974: "The Department has a 'fervent desire' to let the private sector do what it knows best. The reader [of the Federal Register] is 'implored' to understand that the Department is not setting regulations but 'trying to fashion a partnership with the private sector' " (Schmidt 1977:168). Since the failure of that partnership in the late 1970s, there have been no further attempts to develop a national blood system in the United States.[28]

Who Was Guarding the Hen House?

HIV contamination of the blood supply resulting in the deaths of close of half the population of hemophiliacs in France and in the United States was a quintessential "policy tragedy"—"someone [had been] harmed and wrongly so" (Carpenter 2010:74). Finding the culprit is invariably a first step in redressing harm, and much of our story will be about attributions—and deflections—of responsibility for this tragedy. Before launching into those narratives, however, it will be useful to unravel—insofar as possible—and directly compare the location of responsibility for oversight of each country's blood system—in theory and in practice—during the critical period of the early 1980s. France's political and geographical centralization and the relative

---

[28] For a brief description of the current system, largely unchanged from the 1970s, see Mulcahy, *Toward a Sustainable Blood Supply in the United States* published by the Rand Corporation in 2016.

fragmentation of the United States' political system make it easy to assume that oversight of their blood systems was correspondingly centralized (France) and fragmented (United States). The reality—as the foregoing organizational histories may have suggested—was more complicated.

It was not until immediately after the end of the Second World War—and at about the same time—that the French and American governments took official notice of a new and rapidly expanding enterprise centered on the collection and supply of human blood for therapeutic purposes.[29] Both countries began accrediting blood centers in the late 1940s; licenses were issued in France by the Ministry of Health and in the United States by the National Institutes of Health until 1972 and subsequently by the Food and Drug Administration (FDA).[30] Regulation of transfusion centers in France was codified in 1952, as noted earlier: the principal requirements were physician direction, nonprofit status, and careful attention to the health and well-being of donors.[31] Administrative responsibility for oversight of the French blood system was formally located within the Ministry of Health in the Direction Générale de la Santé (DGS);[32] medical oversight was the responsibility of the Comité Consultative de Transfusion Sanguine (CCTS), the majority of whose members were directors of the larger blood centers. *In sharp contrast with the United States (see below), human blood was not classified as a drug and did not fall under France's regime for the regulation of prescription drugs* (Chauveau 2011:186).[33] Despite ongoing criticism (from within) and efforts to reform what at least some experts regarded as an archaic, essentially feudal, system of governance, the organizational structure of the French blood system *"remained practically unchanged [from the 1950s] until the early 1990s"* (Chauveau 2007:23; see also Blin and Bestaux 1971, Hermitte 1996, emphasis added).

---

[29] Our principal sources for this comparison are Beaud 1999, Hermitte 1996, Chauveau 2007 (France); Carpenter 2010, IOM 1995, Starr 2002 (United States).

[30] Licenses were issued in the United States to blood banks engaged in interstate commerce (buying and selling blood across state lines). Regulation of purely local blood banks relied on the basic Food, Drug and Cosmetics Act of 1938.

[31] Details of regulation were strongly influenced by France's organized donor associations (Chauveau 2007). Their primary interest was in the protection of donors, not recipients.

[32] The Direction Générale de la Santé (DGS) is the administrative arm of the French Ministry of Health responsible for public health (including the blood supply). Historically, it has been the weakest arm of the Ministry, sidelined by much larger and better financed sections responsible for personal health services, social security, and hospitals.

[33] France's donor association was powerfully opposed to the classification of blood as a *médicament* (drug). Following the blood crisis and under pressure from the European Union, human blood was reclassified as a *médicament* in 1992 and placed under the same regulatory regime as other pharmaceutical products.

In the United States, "The federal government regulates blood banking [and] monitors the safety and efficacy of blood products" (Office of Technology Assessment 1985, cited in IOM 1995:41). It accomplishes this through "two separate but overlapping statutes, one governing 'biologics' and one governing 'drugs' " (IOM 1995:47).

> The biologics law requires that any 'virus, therapeutic serum, toxin, anti-toxin, or analogous product' be prepared in a facility holding a federal license. A separate law, for food and drugs, includes drugs intended for the 'cure, mitigation, or prevention of disease' and, thus, includes biologics such as blood and blood components or derivatives. *Thus, blood banks and plasma product manufacturers [i.e., fractionators] are also   subject to this drug regulatory process.* (IOM 1995:47, emphasis added)[34]

Implementation of these statutes was (and is) the responsibility of the FDA, an agency of the U.S. government with vast and, indeed, quite remarkable powers, including, "the power to define medical success and shape scientific careers, the power to limit advertising and product claims, the power to govern drug manufacturing, the power to enable drug firms to generate vast riches and the power to chase those same firms from the marketplace, the power to sculpt medical and scientific concepts, and ultimately the power to influence the lives and deaths of citizens" (Carpenter 2010:1; see also Prasad 2012).[35] Within the FDA, responsibility for blood oversight (i.e., of "blood collection, processing, testing, and marketing") was allocated to the Bureau of Biologics (now the Center for Biologics Evaluation and Research [CBER]). The FDA makes extensive use of advisory committees; the Blood Products Advisory Committee (BPAC) was one of four standing committees of the (then) Bureau of Biologics. Its charge was to provide "evaluation of data related to safety, effectiveness, and labeling of blood and blood products and [make] appropriate recommendations to the Secretary, the Assistant Secretary for Health, and the FDA commissioner (IOM 1992, cited in IOM 1995:46). BPAC's composition in the early 1980s included

---

[34] Prior to its amendment in 1970, the Biologics Act (originally passed in 1902) did not specifically include blood products.

[35] The FDA's jealousy of these powers was clearly reflected in its reportedly "furious" response to the CDC's efforts at more proactive action than the FDA was prepared to countenance in response to what the CDC regarded in early 1983 as the high probability of HIV contamination of the blood supply (Bruce Evatt interview, May 10, 2016, retrieved from globalhealthchronicles.com).

blood and plasma organization representatives, scientists, and physicians, but no consumer or patient representatives. BPAC's chair at the time was also the chair of the AABB's Committee on Transfusion Transmitted Diseases.

Both France and the United States had what were, on paper, centralized systems for regulation of the supply and distribution of blood and blood products. In neither case did these systems operate as their formal structures might have led one to expect. In both cases, critical gatekeeping and what organizational theorists would call "sensemaking" power was in the hands of advisory committees largely composed of medical experts representing the regulated entities, the "producers" of blood and blood products.[36] In France, "it was the CCTS that was sovereign, in other words, the transfusion doctors and [blood] center directors. . . . Thus, it was the producers of blood products who decided the characteristics [of these products] and the methods of control" (Chauveau 2011:186). Many of the center directors had held their positions for decades: when he retired in 1984, Jean-Pierre Soulier had directed the Centre National de Transfusion Sanguine (CNTS) for thirty years.[37] Insofar as there was an organizational hierarchy, it stopped at the regional level. The central government had neither the resources, nor the power, nor the will to exercise the authority over the blood system that it indubitably possessed: "*There was no central or national direction*" (Chauveau 2007:94, emphasis added). Commenting in its executive summary on the role in the blood affair of the FDA, the Institute of Medicine Committee to Study HIV Transmission Through Blood and Blood Products stated, "the agency did not adequately use its regulatory authority and therefore missed opportunities to protect the public health" (IOM 1995:7).

---

[36] Abolafia's description of "sensemaking" by the U.S. Federal Open Market Committee ("the Fed") applies equally well to the process undergone by these advisory committees confronted with the uncertainties of AIDS: "Members of an elite policymaking committee engage in hours of deliberation trying to extract the salient cues in that situation, develop a shared narrative that characterizes [makes sense of] the situation, and match that narrative with a policy that seems appropriate" (2020:9). We will have much more to say in later chapters about the beliefs that shaped each country's shared narrative.

[37] We call attention, once again, to the fact that CNTS's name—Centre National de Transfusion Sanguine—is highly misleading. CNTS was the largest of seven regional blood centers, serving Paris and the surrounding area; it engaged in fractionation to produce blood products; and it was tasked by the government with certain special missions, including importation of blood products from abroad. CNTS was neither "national" in organizational scope nor was it a government agency.

Comparative Constructions:
Blood, Technology, and Morality

The divergent trajectories followed by France and the United States in the production of blood and blood products for the civilian population following the Second World War do not in and of themselves account for how each country interpreted and responded to contamination of the blood supply in the 1980s. These histories were nevertheless critical in setting the stage, creating opportunities for political actors in France to cry betrayal and demand not only compensation but also retribution, political opportunities that *simply did not exist* in the United States. The larger political context, government policies of rapid industrialization and modernization in France and of neoliberalism and deregulation in the United States, shaped political opportunities for the amplification of crisis in important ways, and we will return to these contextual effects at a later point. Our focus here is on how national differences in the meanings of blood were constructed (and manipulated) over time and employed in the ongoing calculations of political actors.

America's love affair with technology and embrace of market-based interpretations of and solutions to societal problems are hardly original observations. But the blood narrative allows these cultural traits to stand out with particular clarity—and with intriguing twists—in the light shed by comparison with France. We noted earlier that in American eyes blood had no value absent the technology that recreated it for human use: "Some wish to view blood as a unique human resource to which dollar value cannot realistically be ascribed. *The real value is in the technology* required to take the raw blood from the donor and process it into the form needed by the patient" (Schmidt 1977:164, emphasis added). As head of the NIH Blood Bank, a member of the National Academy of Sciences (NAS) committee to evaluate the blood supply and of the ABC, Schmidt was a major player in the blood politics of the late 1960s and 1970s in the United States; his words in the eyes of his French counterparts would have amounted to sacrilege (whether or not they subscribed to his views). From the French perspective, "irrespective of how it is manipulated and how far it is removed from its origin, blood retains the imprint . . . of its humanity" (Hermitte 1996:107). Retrospectively, French hemophiliacs were identified as the *victims*, not the beneficiaries, of technology. Upon his installation, the director of a commission to oversee their compensation stated, "technological societies have a moral debt to individuals who by chance become the sacrificial victims of progress from which others benefit" (cited in Hermitte 1996:329). In retrospective analyses of the blood affair in France, Hermitte refers to the actions of blood bankers as "technological delinquency" and Fillion questions the value of medical "progress." In sharp contrast, prominent American analysts (and even some American hemophiliacs) concluded their narratives of these events with optimistic visions of patients walking happily into the sunrise of a yet more biotechnologized future (i.e., blood factor genetically engineered to be free of the dangers inherent in human blood) (Resnik 1999, White 2010, Pierce oral history interview, 1990). Technology had no downside.

Construction of blood as a moral object inseparable from its human origins emerged very quickly in France following the second world war. That construction was promoted, and sustained by highly organized, politically connected blood donors active on the local and national level and militant on behalf of voluntary donation and absence of profit from blood. Local transfusion centers depended on donor associations for financial and material support, and the government depended on donors to ensure the national blood supply.[38] In sharp contrast, the meanings attributed to blood in the United States were as fragmented and contested as the arrangements for its supply. It was only a few years after the Conseil d'Etat declared human blood to be totally outside the market that the FTC ruled it a commodity and subject to all the laws of the marketplace. That ruling did not stand, blood was ultimately ruled to be a "service," not a commodity, and by the mid-1970s whole blood donations in the United States had become almost entirely voluntary. None of these policies grew from a newfound commitment to the "moralization" of blood.

The force behind U.S. blood policies as they consolidated in the 1970s was not blood donors—no donor organizations comparable to those in France existed in the United States—but organized medicine as represented by the AMA and the AABB.

A combination of widely shared ethical principles with government financial constraints and blood donor activism led to the rejection of commodification in France; in the United States, it was the threat of product liability. The symbolic significance of blood in France and the economic interests of American doctors, hospitals, and blood banks in avoiding legal liability for

[38] We will return to this point, but it is important to emphasize that this framing of blood engaged substantial economic and political as well as ideological interests.

toxic blood worked to the same end of powerful political opposition to the (formal and/or legal) commodification of blood. Similarly, arguments for *voluntary* donation in the United States were not couched in moral terms— and certainly not in appeals to solidarity—but in the dangers to health posed by paid (and, by implication, economically deprived) donors.

The economics of blood are complicated. There are costs (and potential profits) at every link in the chain from donation to transfusion and/or injection (in the case of blood products). Hospitals and blood banks may find themselves lacking sufficient blood of a particular type or with a surfeit, leading to elaborate networks of exchange with, again, attendant costs. Blood was bought and sold in both countries, often profitably. The abrupt discovery of those costs and that profit—so contrary to the long-standing mystification of blood in France—goes some way to account for the amplitude of the reaction when blood was found to be—in fact—a marketable and marketed commodity.

PART I
HIV/BLOOD STORIES

The next three chapters under the broad label "Blood Stories" are crisis narratives. They tell the stories of HIV contamination of the blood supply, of how it became a full-blown political crisis in France (and not in the United State), and of the social mobilization of the afflicted (principally hemophiliacs but in France transfusion recipients as well).

3

Act I—Before the Storm, 1981–1985

France

Prelude

The French blood crisis was not a single, highly visible, clearly time-delimited event—a hurricane, an earthquake, or even the storming of the Bastille. Nor was the crisis—this "rupture" in human affairs—the infection and subsequent death of many hundreds of French hemophiliacs and transfusion recipients, however horrific these occurrences may have been. The crisis was produced by an accumulation of evidence—and, more significantly, of "symbolic constructions" of that evidence—purporting to demonstrate that French authorities knew of those infections and deaths, knew they were caused by HIV-contaminated blood, concealed that knowledge, and failed to take ap-propriate action. Reconstruction of when and how the French blood affair emerged from the political shadows to be proclaimed as a national crisis is made difficult not only by the passage of time but also by the intense in-vestment in one or another characterization of this event by many of its chroniclers.

The earliest accounts in time were from physicians and scientists who treated AIDS patients before they knew they were AIDS patients and who pioneered the discovery of what caused this mysterious and fatal disease, *"un virus étrange qui vient d'ailleurs"*—a strange virus that comes from afar (Rozenbaum et al. 1984, Leibowitch 1984). Both Rozenbaum, the cli-nician, and Leibowitch, the immunologist, recognized the possibility of blood transmission, but theirs were narratives of medical mysteries and sci-entific achievements, only secondarily of the dangers to patients dependent on blood. The first "official" blood story (September 1991) was by Michel Lucas, then the Inspector General of Social Affairs, tasked by health min-isters in the immediate wake of Casteret's bombshell to say what actually

The Social Production of Crisis. Constance A. Nathanson and Henri Bergeron, Oxford University Press.
© Oxford University Press 2023. DOI: 10.1093/oso/9780197682487.003.0003

"happened" ("just the facts").[1] The Lucas report was light on text and heavy on appended documents. It was followed a year later by an outraged report from the French Senate (then dominated by conservatives) limning a history of secrecy and betrayal (Sourdille and Huriet 1992). The trial in 1992 of four French health officials accused of complicity in the contamination of hemophiliacs and transfusees produced its own story of malfeasance and wrongdoing (Greilsamer 1992). These "official" narratives from different arms of the French government were quickly followed by an equally outraged history (elaborating on her earlier article in *L'Événement du jeudi*) from the journalist, Anne-Marie Casteret, published in 1992, the same year as the Senate report. In 1993, the Assemblée Nationale published its own "official" report, far more neutral in tone from that of the Senate and largely ignored. Later on, there were memoirs from the various actors in this drama (some exculpatory, some reflections on the policy process) and scholarly accounts from social historians, legal scholars, and sociologists. The accumulation of accusatory and exculpatory narratives is an important part of our story, and we will return to these narratives—and the picture of crisis and scandal they paint—in later chapters. For the immediate purpose of describing events of the period, 1981–1985, we rely on contemporary documents along with several detailed histories of the period in question.[2]

Marked differences between France and the United States in this period were (1) the initial absence in France of any epidemic surveillance infrastructure comparable to the CDC capable of early recognition and monitoring of the epidemic; (2) the "othering" of AIDS as of foreign—and, in particular, American—origin; (3) the presence in France, and absence in the United States, of a large, nationwide, and highly mobilized association of blood donors

---

[1] The Inspection Générale des Affaires Sociales (IGAS) is the French government's internal audit, evaluation, and inspection office for health, social security, employment and labor policies and organizations under the general title of "social affairs."

[2] Principal sources for the period, 1981–1982, are the works of Rozenbaum and Leibowitch cited above; Michel Setbon's sociologically inflected history of blood screening in France, Great Britain, and Sweden; Pouvoirs Contre SIDA (1993); and oral history interviews with members of the French Working Group on AIDS conducted by Randy Shilts in 1984 and deposited in the San Francisco Public Library. A major source for the period 1983–1985 are detailed records (meeting minutes, memos) drawn from IGAS's 1992 investigation of blood collected in prisons and deposited in the French National Archives (FNA, Box 19930245-1[CAB 639]). Sources also include (in addition to Setbon) the in-depth study by historian Sophie Chauveau, embodied in the 900-page thesis submitted for her *Habilitation*, "Du don au marché: Politiques du sang en France, années 1940-années 2000" (2007), later published in part as *L'Affaire du Sang Contaminé* (2011); *Le Sang et le Droit* by Marie-Angèle Hermitte (1996); and thirty primary documents (reports, correspondence) dating from 1983 to 1987 submitted as part of the 1991 IGAS report *Transfusion Sanguine et SIDA en 1985*, by Michel Lucas (the Lucas report).

routinely represented at the policy table; and (4) the absence in France, and presence in the United States, of a politicized network of gay organizations in a position to insert themselves into medical/scientific deliberations at the national level on a concerted response to a new and lethal disease. We will argue that the different trajectories of gay activism in the two countries were of critical importance to the difference in their blood stories; here we briefly survey the complex landscape of gay activism in France as it existed in the early 1980s.[3]

The election to the French presidency in 1981 of François Mitterrand—the same year that the first cases of what would come to be known as AIDS were reported by CDC—marked a sharp dividing line in the history of gay organization in France. After a twenty-year period of mostly intellectual discussion fragmented along philosophical and political lines, French homosexuals came together politically in the mid-1970s to demand the repeal of legislation that institutionalized discrimination against gays and gay-oriented cultural products (books, magazines, newsletters, etc.). A period of political action—modeled to some degree on their American counterparts—ensued and was successful: among Mitterrand's first actions was to have these laws repealed. The outcome was a marked shift in the gay organizational landscape. On the one hand, "the most openly political French gay organizations lost steam" (Broqua 2020:15). On the other hand, far from demobilizing gays altogether, the disappearance of unity forged under political pressure led to organizational growth and diversification. But it was a highly apolitical growth focused on the cultivation of identities, lifestyles, and "spaces" for gay community. The absence of dialogue between this community and French health authorities is strongly suggested by the comment of a French epidemiologist expert on AIDS: "You [in the United States] have people who are working in gay associations. There is nothing like that in France. . . . The word gay community had absolutely no sense in France. You have a lot of people who think themselves like that, as gay men, or gay women, but I don't think there is a community" (DGS epidemiologist, Shilts Archives 1984).

Early Warnings, 1981–1983

Writing in 1984, Willy Rozenbaum reflected that he was one of the first doctors in France to "admit the reality of AIDS . . . due to an extraordinary

---

[3] Our principal sources are Pinell 2002, Prearo 2014, Broqua 2020.

coincidence. The very same day that I received the *MMWR* (of June 5, 1981) from Atlanta, a French patient came to see me. He had all the symptoms described in American patients. And like them, he was homosexual. In August 1981, after much uncertainty, the diagnosis was formally established" (Rozenbaum et al. 1984:18). Among the first French cases to come to clinical attention, however, were not gay men but individuals whose most noteworthy characteristic was African origin or recent residence in Africa. Two of these cases were women, one was a man.[4] As additional cases accumulated, a small group of clinicians, joined by two public health physicians from the Direction Générale de la Santé (DGS), formed the French Working Group on AIDS (Association de recherche sur le sida [ARSIDA]).[5] Three things about this group are important to note. First, they read regularly and relied heavily on medical literature published in the United States. Second, they began very quickly to communicate directly and establish collaborative relationships with American colleagues, particularly at the CDC. Third, as described and documented by Rozenbaum himself and by multiple later observers (e.g., Shilts 1987, Seytre 1993, Setbon 1993), not only did these individuals occupy marginal positions in the French medical hierarchy but also work on AIDS was itself marginalized, framed as a small number of cases among stigmatized individuals:

> Most of the people around us didn't believe in this disease with its sexual connotations. Our Director General never wanted to recognize that it was a public health problem. He thought we talked about it entirely too much, that yes, the disease existed, but that was enough. (Public health specialist in DGS). (Setbon 1993:50)

Young, relatively inexperienced, and without important institutional roles or connections either in the major Paris hospitals or the health administration, Rozenbaum's group had few financial or laboratory resources.[6] They were eager to pursue the hypothesis of a viral origin for AIDS (suggested to them by the Africa connection) but at first could not find a virologist willing to

---

[4] The first cases in hemophiliacs in the United States were not reported by CDC's *MMWR* until July 16, 1982.

[5] In labeling this group we use their translation of its name from French to English (see, e.g., Barré-Sinoussi 1983). The group was formed in February 1982 (French immunologist, Shilts Archives, 1984).

[6] ARSIDA received some support from the DGS including from an epidemiologist on the DGS staff.

work with them (Setbon 1993:50, Seytre 1993). They were successful in the fall of 1982 in engaging the interest of Luc Montagnier and his team at the Pasteur Institute. Relatively quickly, by February 1983, Montagnier's team isolated the virus; the results were published in *Science* on May 20, 1983. To the surprise of Montagnier and the Working Group, this discovery received relatively little scientific or public attention in France. In the United States, after the initial publication in *Science*, the Pasteur Institute's discovery was essentially buried.

Reasons for indifference on the part of both the French medical establishment and—inextricably connected—the relevant political authorities are worth recounting in some detail, since this analysis provides important context for the blood crisis that followed. Sitting at the interface between the technical "administrative" world and the "political" public visible world, the most powerful actor in the French political landscape is the ministerial cabinet (Suleiman 1974, Setbon 1993). In the case of the health ministry, this power was historically reinforced by the cabinet's independent access to an alternative source of "technical" advice, that of the elite medical establishment.[7] And so, in the case of AIDS, information and counsel arrived at the cabinet through two channels of highly unequal status, legitimacy, and credibility: elite physicians advising inaction and marginalized "agitators" associated with the disrespected DGS:

> At first it wasn't a political question, an infectious disease, but it became one very quickly. Right away, people were taking about the "gay syndrome": that marginalized the problem right off the bat. Why should we be interested in homosexuals? It was their fault. After, it seemed obvious that those who were interested in it must be homosexuals! (Cabinet member, 1983). (Setbon 1993:58)

Linked to the perception of AIDS as a "gay" disease was its framing as an "American" disease: "People who saw patients were excited. For others it was a curiosity from the United States" (French immunologist, Shilts Archives 1984). In an article published on March 22, 1983, the conservative daily newspaper *Le Figaro* minced no words in identifying AIDS's American provenance, at the same time alerting readers that AIDS may have jumped not

---

[7] Chauveau states that Mitterrand's Socialist government's initial appointment of a Communist (Jacques Roux) to head the DGS was indicative of the DGS' "second rank" status (2007:595).

only its geographical but also its sexual boundaries: "For the past three years, AIDS was a 'gay' syndrome, an American disease . . . [an] object of scientific curiosity rather than alarm, limited to small communities in San Francisco and New York." But now there were "already nearly 40 cases in France." "More worrisome . . . the syndrome has spilled over from the homosexual milieu. It has been established that the virus in question can be transmitted by blood transfusions" (cited in Strazulla 1993:65). Exuding reassurance, the director of the Centre National de Transfusion Sanguine (CNTS; the Paris-centered blood bank) is quoted in this same article as saying that the risks of contamination through blood products are much less in France than in the United States because French blood donors are *bénévoles* (voluntary) and 90 percent of blood products consumed are produced in France (Strazulla 1993:68).[8] Recognition of AIDS as a public health problem would have disrupted existing elite medical agendas and funding allocations; its identification with marginalized agitators and with the United States made it easy for the cabinet to disregard when decisions about resource allocation were made.

It took the international media furor over Robert Gallo's "rediscovery" of the AIDS virus in 1984 for the French authorities to finally pay attention:

> It was necessary to wait until the discovery of the virus by the *Institut Pasteur* was rediscovered in the USA by Gallo in April 1984 for people to believe it. The Prime Minister made his first statement on AIDS in May 1984, that is after the statement by the American Secretary of Health. (Member of the Working Group). (Setbon 1993:63)

Recognition of AIDS came about for two reasons, neither of them to do with its importance as a public health problem. First, isolation of the virus opened up important industrial/commercial opportunities given the potential market for a blood-screening test for its detection. Second, the danger to the blood supply—previously recognized by a handful of specialists, including Montagnier who had earlier tried to bring it to authorities' attention—had now moved to front and center. It was publicized in the popular press and became the hook that Montagnier and members of the Working Group used

---

[8] CNTS data cited by Chauveau indicates that this was a significant exaggeration. In 1983, over half of the AHF (anti-hemophilia factor) produced by CNTS was imported (Chauveau 2011:56). Whether over half the AHF *distributed* by CNTS was imported is not entirely clear but strongly implied by Chauveau's analysis. Writing in retrospect, the former director of CNTS, Jean Pierre Soulier, stated that as early as 1982 he urged hemophiliacs to switch to cryoprecipitates made from much smaller numbers of French donors, but he was ignored (Soulier 1992).

to pull the government into engaging with AIDS. What had been perceived as a threat to homosexuals alone was suddenly transformed into a threat to the general population, with the distinction read as one between "voluntary" and "involuntary" risk-taking. From the political perspective—which was the ministerial perspective—involuntary risk-taking was morally insupportable and demanded public political action:

> I think it's mostly a moral problem because people think there is some injustice in AIDS cases linked to blood transfusion because they think that if you have some surgery or if you have a blood transfusion after a traffic accident, or something like that, you're not responsible for getting the virus. But if you're gay or if you're a drug addict, if you had been to Africa and had some sexual contact with prostitutes, you are responsible for getting the virus. (DGS epidemiologist, Shilts Archives 1984)

The actions that were taken—blood screening and heat treatment of blood products, announced publicly by the prime minister in the summer of 1985—were narrowly conceived and did not entail (nor were they in response to) wider social or political mobilization against AIDS. In a 1984 interview with Randy Shilts, Daniel Defert, founder of AIDES (the principal French NGO fighting AIDS) commented on the government response: "I would say the public powers were not prepared for the situation (i.e., the numbers of patients and the massive disease burden of AIDS). . . . In the French press the problem has been presented either as a gay problem, but mainly as a scientific problem. And with Pasteur everybody was saved, and everybody was expecting some miracle from Pasteur" (Defert interview, Shilts Archives 1984).

Muddled Policy, 1983–1985

Almost all major blood policy decisions in France during the period, 1983–1985, were made by a small body of elite blood bankers, the Commission consultative de la transfusion sanguine (CCTS, or the "Consulting Committee"), composed of "the most influential . . . transfusion doctors," many of them heads of regional blood centers (Chauveau 2011:35). Also represented on the CCTS was the French blood donor federation as well as the DGS.[9] The

---

[9] To our knowledge, the AFH (Association Française des Hémophiles) was not represented on the CCTS.

latter, nominal authority over the blood system, had very little influence over the Consulting Committee's decisions. We briefly trace those decisions and then examine in more detail the particularities of the context in which each decision arose. These same decisions—interpreted in retrospect as at best, incompetent, and at worst, betrayal and even murder—became in 1991–1992 the driver of the *crise de sang*. Our account of these decisions relies insofar as possible on documents produced within a few days of the events in question.[10]

In the spring of 1983, alerted by news of AIDS infection among hemophiliacs in the United States and Spain and by actions taken by the FDA (March 24, 1983) to alert American blood banks of the need for some form of donor selection, CCTS requested an up-to-date report on links between transfusion and AIDS.[11] The report was drafted by physicians and scientists on the staff of the CNTS, located in Paris and the largest—and most influential—of France's blood banks Its content was ambiguous in the extreme, reflected in the discussion that surrounded its presentation on June 9, 1983.[12] On the one hand, the authors stated, "to our present knowledge, there is no evidence for risk of AIDS transmission by [blood] transfusion in France." On the other hand, given the seriousness of the disease and the absence of a specific test, they recommended the institution of blood donor selection based on the same categories proposed by the FDA (see fn.1). They also recommended that hemophiliacs limit their use of commercial (imported) blood products in favor of French manufactured products and that heat treatment of these products should be explored. Discussion of the report revealed, first, disagreement on whether AIDS was transmitted by blood at all (the chair of the CCTS stated there was "no formal proof of AIDS transmission by blood transfusion" [see footnote 12]) and, second, profound discomfort at the idea of questioning potential blood donors. Nevertheless, the Commission appointed a subgroup (drawn primarily from CNTS)

---

[10] In memoirs written after the crisis, several of the major participants wrote their accounts of the events we describe below.

[11] In a letter dated May 4, 1983, Michel Garretta, then the *directeur-adjoint* of CNTS, called the FDA's actions to the attention of his staff. Although the FDA had merely recommended "donor education" on AIDS symptoms and risk factors for AIDS (homosexual or bisexual men with multiple partners, injection drug users, Haitian immigrants, and sexual partners of persons belonging to these risk groups along with the statement that these individuals "should refrain from giving blood"), Garretta appears to have read this as, and recommended to his staff, donor *selection* on the basis of an interrogation of the prospective donor (CAB 639 [19930245/1], May 4, 1983).

[12] Our source for this discussion is the *procès verbale* (PV) (minutes) of the CCTS meeting on June 9, 1983 (CAB 639 [19930245/1] June 9, 1983).

to draft a "circular" on donor selection to be distributed by the DGS to the country's blood banks and signed by its director, Jacques Roux.[13]

Background information for the "AIDS and transfusion" report was largely drawn from the United States. No cases of blood transfusion AIDS had been reported in France; the authors described six cases of "immuno-logic abnormalities" in young hemophiliacs but stated these symptoms could well be due to something other than AIDS. The most striking aspect of this report and the discussion that surrounded it—one that every commentator on this event has remarked upon—is the belief among CCTS members that France was protected against blood-transmitted AIDS by its national boundaries and, more specifically, by the fact that French blood was "benevolent" unpaid blood, altruistically donated by persons who were, almost by definition, healthy in body and mind (i.e., not homosexual or drug users). "In the United States, it is the paid donors that are the problem" (Ducos, chair of CCTS, March 24, 1983]). FNA, Box 19930245-1(CAB 639). AIDS was framed by much of the French press in this period as an "American" disease (Herzlich and Pierret 1988). It was a short step to attribute AIDS that made its way into French veins as carried by "American" blood.[14]

A second, more subtle, question concerned the impact on CNTS's position of its major investment in fractionation. Jean-Pierre Soulier, then the director of CNTS and a major figure for many years in the French blood community, suggested that physicians should be urged to switch their hemophiliac patients away from factor concentrates to less risky blood products. Noting the silence of his CNTS colleagues on this point, Chauveau speculated their reluctance was due to CNTS having recently reorganized to become a major producer of just such concentrates.[15] Setbon was more explicit: "The AIDS risk that weighed heavily on the blood transfusion system, was cleverly transformed into a resource for reducing the system's position of dependence on the international market" (Setbon 1993:106). National self-sufficiency in blood as the answer to AIDS was supported by the Council of Europe as well: "Avoid the importation of blood products from countries

---

[13] As noted earlier, the DGS was itself a weak link in France's healthcare system with no obvious counterpart in the American healthcare landscape. Within the DGS, the office responsible for oversight of the blood system consisted of a single person, a non-physician without a strong position or connections.

[14] Our sources include multiple references to importation of American blood products; we have been unable to determine in what amounts or the percentage of total products consumed.

[15] Unfortunately for the fortunes of CNTS, its concentrates were not heat treated, so their production facilities for AHF were outdated almost as soon as they were put in place.

with high risk populations as well as products from paid donors" (Council of Europe 1983). The economic/financial implications of blood policy decisions—in other words, how might a policy of national self-sufficiency in blood affect the finances of CNTS—were a constant thread throughout French policy deliberations in real time, not only as they were reinterpreted in the early 1990s.

Soulier—to a much milder degree, the Donald Francis of the French policy process—stated in the course of the Consulting Committee's June 9, 1983 deliberations: "The Americans have already taken certain precautions; France should also take action to stop this epidemic now" (FNA, Box 19930245-1[CAB 639], June 9, 1983).[16] Striking to an American observer is the French reliance for information and guidance not only on American data but also on American policy, down to the specific categories of blood donors to be singled out for possible exclusion. At the time of which we write, the French government had no visible and even marginally legitimate source of scientific information on the emerging epidemic comparable to CDC in the United States. Minutes of an early Consulting Committee meeting (March 24, 1983) point to a presentation by the French Working Group on AIDS, but no evidence that the latter's insistence on the probability of AIDS transmission through the blood supply was given more than a hearing. The FDA's recommendations, released on that very same day, appear to have received greater attention. When the Consulting Commission wanted reviews of the latest scientific and epidemiologic information on AIDS, it requested these data from its own members, principals of the largest French blood banks. French blood policy decisions in the early 1980s were channeled through a single—far from disinterested—source of information on the character and spread of AIDS. The French Working Group was sidelined, and the DGS had no scientific capability independent of the transfusion system itself and, more specifically, of CNTS.[17]

The "circular" on donor selection was issued on June 20, 1983, only a few days after the meeting of June 9, drafted by the same individuals who wrote the report that recommended it, with the addition of an epidemiologist

---

[16] Soulier put his money where his mouth was. As of May 1983, a month before action was recommended by the DGS, he independently put in place a questionnaire to CNTS's prospective blood donors, asking explicitly about homosexual sex with multiple partners, injection drug use, and Caribbean origin. He was attacked by the French press as homophobic and racist (Muller 2004).

[17] The United States had vastly more and much less narrowly sourced data, partially—but only partially—accounting for the FDA's March 20, 1983, letters to the American blood community that served as a model for the French "circular" to follow two months later.

from the DGS. It was transmitted to its intended audience of "blood bank physicians" by a rather circuitous route, through the *préfet* (the central government official) in each of France's 101 *départements* to the departmental (DDASS) and regional (DRASS) public health authorities, and from there to the individual blood banks.[18] The circular (again, much discussed in French commentary on the blood crisis) played down the risk of AIDS through blood transfusion, describing it variously as "suspected but not established" and as "minimal" in France. Its list of categories "at risk" was identical to those earlier (March 24, 1983) identified by the FDA. The circular asks recipients to inform blood donors and their associations of the need to take precautions and to consider, in collaboration with donor associations, how best to adapt the recommended measures to local conditions. It recommends that physicians in charge of blood collection inform blood donors of the risk categories. A sample information sheet was attached, stating that the risk of transmission "is certainly minimal in France," listing the aforesaid categories, and asking the prospective donor to inform the physician if any of this information "concerns you." No questionnaire was suggested, nor did the information ask the donor to refrain from giving blood—simply to tell the doctor.

A survey carried out in the spring of 1984 showed that this circular was essentially a dead letter on arrival, its recommendations followed inconsistently, if at all (Chauveau 2007:678). A memo from the director of a regional blood center to his physicians charged with blood collection explains why: "'Identification' of persons belonging to at risk populations, as requested by the DGS, is in my opinion illusory and could only result in distrust of the respect we must have, and you must always have for every person who comes to offer blood. Therefore, no indelicate questions or derogatory remarks. . . . If you have questions, take the blood and mark it with a special code. Never refuse blood" (dated July 13, 1983, emphasis in original FNA, Box 19930245-1[CAB 639]). Making explicit reference to the "slight application" of this circular, a second more insistent but otherwise similar circular was issued eighteen months later (January 16, 1985), but by that time blood bankers were waiting for or had already put in place the "test."

In the spring of 1984, Margaret Heckler, secretary of the U.S. Department of Health and Human Services, announced the discovery of the AIDS virus

---

[18] DRASS = "Direction Régionale des Affaires Sanitaires et Sociales." DDASS= "Direction Départementale des Affaires Sanitaires et Sociales." This circuitous route may explain why some blood banks later claimed never to have received the circular.

by Robert Gallo. "France did not wake up," said Montagnier, "until the big media splash made by the Americans in 1984" (Setbon 1993:64). Setbon argues, plausibly we believe, that the wake-up call resulted less from recognition of a major public health problem than of a major industrial and commercial opportunity.[19] Discovery of the virus opened up the possibility of a test for its presence in human blood, a test with an enormous potential market. In the interview cited above, Montagnier went on to say that he met with the minister of industry almost immediately after the Gallo announcement and from there proceeded to make necessary arrangements for the mass production of what would become the "Pasteur" HIV test.

Recognition of danger to the blood supply, the financial implications (in France) of testing donated blood on a national scale, and what became a competition between the Pasteur test and an American test (Abbott) that beat Pasteur to the market triggered the French government's engagement with AIDS. In announcing the institution of mandatory testing on June 19, 1985, Prime Minister Laurent Fabius told the French National Assembly, "with AIDS, we are confronted by an epidemic that might spread. Transmission by blood transfusion represents the danger that AIDS, which at present affects only a limited number of persons, spreads more widely in the population. That is why . . . we must act" (Lucas 1991, #21). Official notice of mandatory testing of "each blood donation" was published in the *Journal Official* on July 23, 1985, to go into effect on August 1; a separate notice, published on the same day, announced that as of October 1, 1985, only heat-treated blood products would be reimbursed by the health insurance system, effectively cutting off new prescriptions of non-heat-treated products.

Demand for testing among the medical elites of the blood system had built quickly beginning in late 1984 when (1) first noncommercial tests and then the Abbott test became available and (2) data from these tests revealed the extent of HIV contamination of blood drawn on the streets of Paris.[20] These latter results were communicated to colleagues in the blood system and to the DGS in a letter from the director of a Paris blood bank dated January 9, 1985, stating in its first sentence: "The possibility of AIDS transmission by blood transfusion is certain" (Lucas, 1991:#7). Two months later, an epidemiologist

---

[19] In an article published on April 25, 1984, shortly after Heckler's press conference, *Figaro* asked whether the "royalties" stemming from this discovery would be paid in francs or dollars (Herzlich and Pierret 1988:1118). The financial implications of the French-American competition were hardly a secret.

[20] Most blood collection was done from mobile vans.

on the staff of the DGS sent a memo to the director noting, based on additional results from Paris blood banks: "It is likely that all blood products produced from Parisian blood donor pools are contaminated" (Lucas 1991, #11, emphasis in original). What had earlier been merely "suspected," was now made visible and indisputable. Herzlich and Pierret date the entry of AIDS into the French "public space" from the spring of 1985, reflected in an over 500 percent increase from 1984 to 1985 in the number of relevant articles published in six newspapers with a national circulation.[21] "The government's decision to require screening for all blood donors . . . signaled that AIDS was no longer only a private problem of the sick or a professional problem of physicians, but a problem for the State, and would continue from then on to be an object of political attention" (Herzlich and Pierret 1988:1125).

The article by Herzlich and Pierret was published in 1988, three years before eruption of the blood crisis, well before public perspectives on the early years of AIDS in France—and in particular, on the events of 1985—were altered almost beyond recognition. From the distance of three years—using the Lucas report, published in 1991, as a touchstone—the key events of 1985 were first, resolution of the battle of the HIV blood tests between Pasteur and Abbott and, second, the decision by CNTS not to recall contaminated blood products but to distribute contaminated products to already infected hemophiliacs and uncontaminated products to those uninfected ("double distribution"). These decisions—we will return to them below—were made behind closed doors. They were not what preoccupied the French press in 1985. Public fear, even panic, raised by the possibility—articulated by the prime minister himself—that AIDS might spread beyond a few marginalized groups was a central preoccupation accompanied by efforts at reassurance that, at least according to Herzlich and Pierret, had the opposite effect of creating panic. Press attention to "healthy carriers" infected and possibly contagious but not visibly "sick," Rock Hudson's appearance—and death—in Paris, and a much-mediated report of a new AIDS treatment, all contributed to the construction of AIDS as a new and fearsome "social fact."

In the meantime, policy initiatives played out behind the scenes—in the first instance by the government, in the second by principals of the blood system—on two questions central to retrospective interpretations: how to ensure a market for the French (Pasteur) test, and what to do about

---

[21] These newspapers, in order of number of AIDS articles published (from most to least) were *Le Monde, Libération, Le Matin, Le Figaro, Le Quotidien, L'Humanité*.

HIV-contaminated blood products already in clinics, on pharmacy shelves, and in the homes of hemophiliacs. The American (Abbott) test was submitted to French authorities for approval on February 11, 1985, the Pasteur test on February 28. The latter was approved on June 21, within four months of its submission, the former on July 24, a delay of over five months. Internal memos and minutes of ministerial meetings document several reasons for delay: concerns about the cost of mass blood testing, demands for further evaluation of the tests, but the principal reason was that Pasteur lagged behind Abbott, and Abbott had already captured a significant portion of the French market. "The cost of screening didn't faze us. For the authorities, it was not a problem of cost. The delay was because Pasteur wasn't ready" (DGS official, cited in Setbon 1993:118). This reading is supported by interministerial meeting minutes: on May 9, 1985, after considerable discussion including the statement that "Abbott's strategy is to eliminate the French competition," the cabinet of the prime minister requested that Abbott's registration be delayed (*Compte-rendu de la réunion interministérielle tenue le 9 mai 1985* [Lucas 1991 #17]).[22]

CNTS's decision not to recall blood products known to be contaminated has a longer and more complicated history, rooted in irreconcilability between the French blood system's founding myth of benevolence and nonprofit and the mass production and competitive marketing of blood products. CNTS was not merely one of many blood banks in France. It was the first among equals. It encompassed not only blood collection but also clinical, research, and training activities; it was the principal manufacturer of blood products in France (only one other blood bank did fractionation), and it had other specialized responsibilities, including the sole entity with the authority to import blood products. CNTS had operated under massively conflicting pressures for many years before 1985: pressures from the other actors in the blood system—hemophiliacs, the state, other blood banks, organized blood donors—to maintain the appearance of nonprofit while contributing to national self-sufficiency in blood and its derivatives, avoiding importation of "commercial" blood products, supplying hemophiliacs' increasing demand for AHF, keeping abreast of the latest advances in blood technology, and balancing its books. Whatever its success in other respects, CNTS failed to balance its books: a deficit in millions of francs nearly quadrupled between 1980 and 1983 (Chauveau 2011:57). Nevertheless, "whether the goal of national

---

[22] This *compte-rendu* was no. 17 of 31 original documents appended to the Lucas report.

self-sufficiency was achieved (or appeared to be achieved) at the price of accounting acrobatics or conflicts of interest mattered little. Questionable practices in the management of CNTS bothered neither its directors nor the State: it was not until much later, in the context of crisis, that these practices would be attacked" (Chauveau 2011:55).[23]

By the end of 1984, the majority of French blood bankers had become convinced that AIDS transmission through blood products was a fact, that heat treatment was effective in killing the virus, and that the shift to heat-treated AHF was essential (Chauveau 2007:685).[24] Accomplishing this shift within the organizational, ideological, and financial constraints imposed by the French blood system was another matter altogether and took almost a year.[25] In March of 1985, the Consulting Committee (CCTS) put together a working group, AIDS and Blood Transfusion, to provide guidance to the government and the blood community (Lucas 1991:38).[26] The report of this working group—and its tortuous and only partially known trajectory—formed the scaffolding on which the blood crisis six years later was built. Two versions of this report were produced. The first version, presented to the CCTS on May 14, 1985, called for recall of all blood products from HIV-contaminated lots, the replacement of already distributed products with "safe" products, the use of (the much safer) "cryos" if necessary, and the import of heat-treated products (Chauveau 2007:693). The second and final version of the report—submitted to the health minister on May 30 and copied to the DGS—"was significantly different from the one discussed on May 14, specifically with respect to the disposition of blood products that may have been contaminated" (Chauveau 2007:693). The final report offered two choices: do nothing (l'abstention de toute intervention), or "the recall of all unused products and the discontinuation of all product distribution" (Lucas 1991, #15). Import of heat-treated products as an alternative

[23] No doubt adding to the pressure at that time on CNTS generally and Garretta in particular was an ongoing investigation of its organization and finances by Inspection Générale des Affaires Sociales (IGAS) (Rapport n° 850 présenté par Mme le docteur Broyelle et Mme Jeannet, membres de l'IGAS sur le fonctionnement du CNTS, 19 septembre, 1985).

[24] Our use of the word "majority" is based on the language in an "expert" report produced in May 1985 that demonstrates continuing doubts about the efficacy of "foreign" heat-treated blood products (Lucas 1991, #15).

[25] We remind the reader that CCTS was the body of experts providing regulatory oversight to the French blood system. CNTS was the largest French blood bank, headquartered in Paris.

[26] The composition of this "working group" included the same three experts from CNTS that had produced the 1983 report described earlier plus a CNTS immunologist, outside virologists, representatives from other blood banks, the Pasteur Institute, the French federation of blood donors, and the DGS (Lucas 1991:38). The leader of this group was Dr. Bahman Habibi, physician in charge of products distribution at CNTS. The report became known as the "Habibi report."

was mentioned in the final report only to dismiss these "foreign" products as possibly not available in sufficient quantity and anyway of questionable value (Lucas 1991, #15). The working group "was unable to reach agreement on this dilemma." Consequently, it was up to the "national health authorities" to choose between "do nothing" or recall. The report went on to propose an interim policy to fill the gap before French manufactured heat-treated AHF became available: sero-negative hemophiliacs would get imported heat-treated products; sero-positives would continue to receive products that were potentially contaminated. This interim policy was endorsed on two occasions by the French association of hemophiliacs in early May and late June 1985.[27] The final reported submitted on May 30 was accepted without comment by the Ministry of Health and the DGS. It was presented to the June 20, 1985, meeting of the CCTS with, again, no recorded critical comment. There was no scandal in the summer of 1985 (Chauveau 2007:698).[28]

Documents contemporary with the two versions of the "Habibi report" go some way toward accounting for its shifting content. On May 9, 1985, Michel Garretta, the director of CNTS, wrote in the strongest possible terms to the person in the DGS responsible for blood and blood products. Garretta's letter reads as a genuine *cri de coeur*. He began by stating that half of French hemophiliacs were already contaminated and that "it is now of the utmost urgency to stop the spread of this contamination among hemophiliacs and their families" (Lucas 1991:#10). He described the preparations CNTS had made to meet the demand for untreated AHF and stated that project would now be abandoned. He went on to lay out a plan for meeting the challenge of a rapid shift to heat-treated products and—of critical importance—the costs that shift would entail not only in new equipment but also in ensuring a supply of treated blood products to hemophiliacs in the interim before CNTS was fully prepared to manufacture those products itself. "The financial consequences of this urgent strategy are considerable . . . after offering several options for making up these costs this is vital for C.N.T.S., economically it has no other

[27] AFH argued after 1991 that its members had been insufficiently informed. There is some evidence that Garretta orchestrated the association's approval. He met with its president in late April and, Chauveau argues, it was at that meeting that the October 1 date for transition to heat-treated products was set. The October 1 date was approved officially by the ANH on May 10.

[28] The single recorded exception at the time to the bland response of experts and government officials to the conscious distribution of contaminated blood products was the remarkably prescient letter, dated July 5, 1985, to the president of the CCTS from the director of the regional blood center in Toulouse: "It is unacceptable today to continue [distributing contaminated products] on the pretext that French products are not available. . . I am convinced this will be a scandal if the media get hold of it and that transfusion doctors and those who take care of hemophiliacs will be rightly accused of negligence" (Lucas 1991:55–56).

solution" (Lucas 1991, #10). This letter was copied to the principals of CNTS. No answer to this letter from the DGS has been recorded.

On May 29, 1985, a meeting of CNTS's inner circle was convened that included Dr. Garretta along with Dr. Habibi and the other CNTS expert members of the AIDS and Blood Transfusion working group. The "confidential" record of this meeting contained the statement, "all our lots are contaminated" as well as a restatement of their choices as they saw them: (1) recall and end distribution of potentially contaminated products, (2) distribute foreign (heat-treated) blood products to fill the resulting gap in product availability, (3) assume that French heat-treated products will be available soon and in the meantime continue distribution unchanged. The "serious" financial implications of the first and second options were invoked. The meeting minutes contain no record of discussion around the solution that was finally adopted: "No recall of and no discontinuation of finished product distribution, knowing that statistical calculation shows unfortunately that all our pools are currently contaminated. It is up to the government [autorités de tutelle] to accept responsibility for this serious problem and possibly to prohibit us from distributing these products, with the financial consequences that would entail" (Lucas 1991, #18).

"It seems quite clear," argues Chauveau, "that the second version of the expert recommendations was edited to accommodate the specific situation of CNTS," that is, its unique position as the principal manufacturer and sole importer of blood products under circumstances where the financial implications of that position—laid out in Garretta's letter to the DGS—continued to be mystified (and also—to all appearances—rejected by the Ministry of Health). Both Chauveau and Hermitte suggest that Garretta was, himself, so invested in the goal of national self-sufficiency in blood products that reliance, even temporarily, on imported products was personally unacceptable. Chauveau concludes, "the CNTS and its interests continued to dominate choices made by the transfusion system. The contradictions of the French transfusion system appear here in dramatic fashion, where preservation of its façade led to decisions contrary to medical ethics" (2007:694).

United States

"In the first 6–12 months of the epidemic, virtually nobody seemed to care about it. That meant that nobody was opposed to it, nobody was offended by it, and nobody was excited about it, and no one was funding it" (Curran interview, CDC/Emory Archives, February 10, 2016).[29] Curran is referring to the United States, but his description applies equally well to France. In this vacuum of interest and leadership, the critical differences between the two countries were, first, the overwhelming dominance in the United States of the CDC in communicating, identifying, and framing the epidemic and, second, the early, strong, and vocal presence of gay organizations and, in particular gay physicians, in U.S. Public Health Service (PHS) organized bodies to deliberate on a response to the threat of blood contamination.[30] A third key element was the tightly networked structure of relationships among the public health and medical players in this earliest phase of the AIDS/blood threat.

CDC on the Front Line

For at least the first three years of the epidemic—until the virologists took center stage with Gallo's rediscovery of the AIDS virus—the *scientific* narrative of AIDS was almost entirely driven by the CDC both in the United States and internationally. The universe within which this information circulated was very small and highly interconnected. These connections are clearly reflected in (and were, of course, fostered by) the reappearance of the same names and affiliated agencies and organizations of individuals present at those early meetings. They also included—by phone, mail, and occasionally in person—members of what became the tiny French research task force on AIDS (the French Working Group). We divide this period into three stages: 1981–1982, when CDC labeled the constellation of symptoms they were reporting as "Acquired Immune Deficiency Syndrome" (AIDS) and became convinced that these symptoms were caused by a single blood-borne

---

[29] Oral history interviews compiled by CDC's "Global Health Chronicles" project in collaboration with Emory University were an invaluable resource for this work. They are subject to the same cautions we have identified earlier with regard to retrospective recollections, in the case of these interviews between thirty and thirty-four years after the events being recalled. However, where facts are in question we have been able to corroborate almost all of these retrospective accounts with documents contemporary with the events described.

[30] The earliest federally sponsored meetings (1982, January 1983) were initiated by the CDC. The role of the FDA as a sponsoring partner in these meetings is a bit unclear, but it appears to have been consulted. Meetings sponsored by blood banks and by the NHF also included representatives of organized gay physicians. Industry-sponsored meetings did not.

agent; the now famous Atlanta meeting of January 1983; and 1983–1985, when the AIDS threat to the blood supply was recognized and contained.

1981–1982
On July 16, 1982, in its sentinel weekly report to the public health and medical community (*Morbidity and Mortality Weekly Report* [*MMWR*]), the CDC described three cases of pneumocystic pneumonia (PCP) among hemophiliacs, stating that "although the cause of the severe immune dysfunction is unknown, the occurrence among the three hemophilia cases suggests the possible transmission of an agent through blood products." Underlying this cautiously worded statement was "almost complete unanimity in the halls of CDC" that they were confronting a blood-borne infectious agent (Lawrence interview, Resnik Archives, October 11, 1991).[31] This unanimity—carrying conviction (and even passion)—comes through clearly in retrospective interviews with CDC epidemiologists who worked on the AIDS epidemic:[32] "It wasn't until there were three cases reported in people with hemophilia who automatically had received transfusions from hundreds of thousands of people (the perfect canary in the coal mine for a new blood-borne infection) that blood-borne transmission was convincing. Once those three cases of AIDS in persons with hemophilia were well documented by CDC's Dr. Dale Lawrence, then everybody recognized the causative agent of AIDS was likely a virus and in the blood supply" (Curran interview, CDC/Emory Archives, February 10, 2016). Recognition favored the prepared mind, however, and while "we [the CDC] were convinced, the rest of the world wasn't" (Evatt interview, CDC/Emory Archives, May 10, 2016).

Conviction arose in part from the unusual depth of collective scientific background among the CDC's scientific staff that combined epidemiology with infectious diseases, virology, retrovirology, and hematology, but also from the highly networked mode of operation that was characteristic of the CDC: "One of the really good things is that CDC swarms on new problems with the Epidemic Intelligence Service [EIS] and the general mentality of responding to a threat" (Curran 2/10/16 [CDC/Emory Collection]).[33] More

[31] Dale Lawrence was an Epidemic Intelligence Service (EIS) officer with CDC in the early 1980s. His interview is from the Resnik Archives deposited with Columbia University.
[32] The bulk of these interviews were collected as part of the CDC/Emory University oral history project, "The Early Years of AIDS: 1981–1988."
[33] James Curran led the CDC AIDS Task Force from its inception and through its various iterations in nomenclature.

specifically, "We had many connections with doctors [and in the infectious disease community]. Doctors [on the CDC staff] knew people who knew people. We knew people from our Hepatitis B studies in [the gay] community, and then we knew who had requested pentamidine [to treat pneumocystis pneumonia]. So we made these kinds of connections within the first week or so [of June 1981] and made a couple of visits in the first couple of weeks. Then shortly thereafter we dispatched EIS officers to 18 cities to conduct more intensive surveillance in their pathology logs and their infectious disease logs in major hospitals to look for cases" (Curran 2/10/16 [CDC/ Emory Collection]). The CDC had strong connections not only with public health and medical communities that it was able to immediately activate but also within the gay community and, in particular gay physicians, grounded in projects around STDs and hepatitis that long preceded AIDS. The density and positive cast of the CDC's relationships with its public health, hospital, and physician constituencies lay in sharp contrast to the experience of the French AIDS research group in its initial efforts to engage the closed, hierarchically organized world of French medicine: "We weren't competing with anyone, because no one was working on [AIDS]. . . , but also, no one in the institution [hospital] could help us" (Setbon 1993:49).

Convinced that they were dealing with a blood-borne agent, the CDC moved in the summer of 1982 to expand its stakeholder network "to see how serious this potentially could be for the blood system of America and for hemophilia patients in particular" (Lawrence interview, Resnik Archives, October 11, 1991). With the goal of alerting and engaging the blood industry along with its federal partners (the FDA and the NIH), the CDC convened back-to-back meetings, the first on the same day, July 16, 1982, when the three hemophilia cases were announced in the *MMWR*. The cast of characters included (besides CDC staff) representatives of the blood industry,[34] the National Hemophilia Foundation, FDA, NIH, the National Gay Task Force and (at the second meeting on July 27), the New York City Health Department, and the New York InterHospital Study Group on AIDS.[35]

[34] The "blood industry" includes the nonprofits (the American Red Cross and the two principal blood bank organizations [AABB, CCBC] and the for-profits (the industry trade association [American Blood Resources Association] plus the individual manufacturers [Cutter, Baxter, Alpha, Armour]).

[35] With very little variation (occasional additions, few if any subtractions) this same cast was present at all subsequent meetings on the blood supply held in 1982–1983. We will argue that this highly interconnected relationship structure across multiple actors in the blood field was a key element in preventing contamination of the blood supply from becoming a full-scale crisis in the United States (Clemens and Cook 1999).

A positive outcome of these meetings from the CDC's perspective was the adoption of "Acquired Immune Deficiency Syndrome" (AIDS) to name the complex of symptoms they were observing, a move the CDC quite deliberately engineered (see Curran 2/10/16 [CDC/Emory Collection]). In other respects, they were a disappointment: "We received somewhat of a cold shoulder" (Evatt 5/10/16 [CDC/Emory Collection]). Evatt went on to describe each stakeholder's reaction at this early stage:

> The blood banking industry is a very stable industry. Changes occur over long periods of time. They were not interested [in any modifications based on] three cases. . . . The homosexual community were extremely good donors. They thought they were very civic minded in donating blood. . . . In some cities they made up as much of a third of the donors. . . . The blood banking community wasn't interested at all in raising any kind of hassle about the fact that some of their donors may be donating and may be causing this disease. And three patients with hemophilia they felt was no proof at all. The hemophilia community was interested, but—they saw [AHF/Factor VIII] as being a major life-changing event for patients with hemophilia. And to raise the possibility that maybe it was transmitting this new disease, when there were only three cases, it was so rare that they didn't want patients stopping the medicine. They were not interested in hearing of it as a risk either, and there was still no proof. At that point in time, you still had lots of people believing that it was something else causing AIDS. It wasn't really a disease, that it was a reaction to amyl nitrites. The FDA didn't believe it was a disease. They were not particularly interested. (Evatt interview, CDC/Emory Archives, May 10, 2016)

This is a relatively dispassionate account at thirty-five years remove from the events in question. Comments from a blood industry insider—no particular friend to the CDC—make clear that passions at the time ran high: "Let me just tell you [what] I heard from CDC on several occasions in various places. It was phrased slightly differently each time but it was, if you guys don't do something, you won't have a hemophilia problem to deal with because all the hemophiliacs will be dead" (FDA BPAC, 2/7/83).

Atlanta Meeting, January 3, 1983
This standing-room only meeting of "experts"—essentially the same experts present at the July meetings with the addition of transfusion

specialists—called to "formulate recommendations for the prevention of AIDS with special emphasis on possible transmission through blood and blood products," has been frequently and dramatically described (Drake 1983, Shilts 1987, IOM 1995, Bayer 1999).[36] This was a public meeting: the press was invited, and the meeting was reported by the Associated Press and in the *New York Times* (on an inside page) with the headline "Disease Stirs Fear on Blood Supply" (January 6, 1983:B17). There was no effort at concealment—and almost no media follow-up.

From the CDC's perspective, blood transmission was at this point a given, and the purpose of the meeting was to formulate strategies for prevention, specifically rigorous screening of blood donors that included questions on sexual preference and—in the absence of a more specific blood test that waited on discovery of the virus—testing for hepatitis B which, the CDC argued, was relatively cheap and highly correlated with AIDS. Both the premise of a blood-borne infection and the proposed means of prevention were anathema to many of the "experts" present, resulting in the famous image of a frustrated Dr. Donald Francis pounding the table with his fist. In his own words, "the outcome of this . . . meeting was so extraordinary that my quiet self pounded the table. Literally pounded the table!" (Francis 10/13/16 [CDC/Emory Collection]). Despite this frustration—recollected uniformly and in much the same terms by other CDC scientists who were present— Evatt dates "the start of a shift in thinking" from the Atlanta meeting: "That was the beginning, when people began the process of the paradigm shift [away from] thinking this is a gay disease and putting more and more emphasis on blood" (Evatt interview, CDC/Emory Archives, May 10, 2016).

1983–1985

The most immediate result of the Atlanta meeting was a flurry of further meetings and memos back and forth initiated by the National Hemophilia Foundation (NHF) and the blood industry. The gist of these conversations was to raise questions about CDC scientists' competence, motives, and credibility and to oppose their recommendations for protection of the blood supply as unjustified and unnecessary. In comments by members of the FDA's

---

[36] A detailed description, clearly depicting the conflicting interests and absence of consensus that prevailed at that date and time was written by reporter Donald C. Drake and published on the front page of the *Philadelphia Inquirer* one week later, on January 9, 1983, with the title, "The Disease Detectives Puzzle over Methods of Control." The *New York Times* appears to have simply printed the AP report with no by-line and almost no commentary. The danger to the blood supply did not become a major media event at the time, nor was it ever taken up by the Reagan administration.

Blood Products Advisory Committee and by blood industry executives following the January 1983 Atlanta meeting, CDC was accused of

1) exaggerating an earlier epidemic threat (swine flu) with disastrous consequences; 2) needing "a major epidemic to justify its existence"; 3) "getting increasingly involved in areas beyond their area of expertise"; and 4) being anxious "to have a high profile in the press." In short, CDC cannot be trusted "to provide scientific objective, unbiased leadership"; "whenever possible we should try to deflect activity to the NIH/FDA."[37]

In the meantime, simultaneously with its search for cases in the field, the CDC was pursuing the cause of AIDS in its own laboratories: "When you have a suspect new infection, one needs to bring both the lab at CDC and the collaborators outside together as fast as possible to find the bug" (Francis 10/13/16 [CDC/Emory Collection]). Frustrated in their efforts to collaborate with NIH and by the disinterest of the FDA, the CDC found partners among the French Working Group and at the Pasteur Institute where Francis had worked previously.

The IOM report on HIV and the blood supply is subtitled "An Analysis of *Crisis* Decisionmaking" (IOM 1995, emphasis added). This is misleading. Among the principal actors at the time, only the CDC identified the threat to the blood supply as an urgent public health problem. The CDC's voice was muffled by higher-ups in the PHS bureaucracy and discounted by its partner federal agencies (the FDA and the NIH), by the blood industry, and by the NHF. Buried in a memo by one of its members on a meeting of the blood product manufacturers' professional association in March 1983 is a comment on a "3 hour presentation" by a CDC scientist (Bruce Evatt), labeled by the memo's author "some items of interest for the record": The "scientist" (Evatt) "expects 50% [of the hemophilia population] to come down with AIDS" (reproduced in Kuhn 1995).[38] As late as December 1983, a PHS flyer, "Facts About AIDS," refers to the "occurrence of AIDS" "in a few

---

[37] These quotations are drawn from internal memos and recorded discussions by blood industry insiders in the period immediately following the CDC meeting on January 4, 1983. Sources are as follows, in the same order as above: American Red Cross internal memo, February 8, 1983; Blood Industry Strategy Meeting, January 14, 1983; Joseph Bove at closed meeting of BPAC, February 7, 1983; and American Red Cross internal memo, February 8, 1983. These items are available in multiple overlapping archival sources, many of them published. See, e.g., IOM 1995; Kuhn 1995.

[38] The "most significant item" to come out of the meeting from this individual's perspective was a draft of soon-to-be-published FDA recommendations "to decrease the risk of transmitting infectious diseases from plasma donors" (reproduced in Kuhn 1995).

hemophilia patients" (U.S. National Archives [Curran Archives]). The NHF via its flyer *Hemophilia NewsNotes* continued through at least 1984 to recommend continued use of Factor VIII (AHF). Not only was there no publicly visible "crisis" in decision-making on the blood supply but the principal stakeholders also made every effort to ensure against a crisis emerging.[39]

The first official recommendation to protect the blood supply was published on March 4, 1983, in *MMWR*: "As a temporary measure, members of groups at increased risk for AIDS should refrain from donating plasma and/or blood." This statement was signed by the CDC, FDA, and NIH and was prefaced by an acknowledgment that while "the National Gay Task Force, the National Hemophilia Foundation, the American Red Cross, the American Association of Blood Banks, the Council of Community Blood Centers, the American Association of Physicians for Human Rights, and others . . . agree that steps should be implemented to reduce the potential risk of transmitting AIDS through blood products . . . [they] differ in the methods proposed to accomplish this goal." (*MMWR* 32 [83], March 4, 1983). This statement was followed on March 24, 1983, by recommendations for implementation from the FDA directed to the blood industry, recommendations that did not include the mandatory donor deferral of high-risk groups and surrogate blood testing proposed by the CDC in their original draft. As recounted by Bruce Evatt: "A firestorm hit, because we [the CDC] were overstepping our bounds once more, even more than the January 4th meeting. The FDA was absolutely furious. Absolutely furious. They flew down and met with Walt Dowdle, who was my boss and Jim Curran's boss." And the recommendations were "watered down" (Evatt interview, CDC/Emory Archives, May 10, 2016).

Once this flurry of activity had passed, blood safety policies, as the IOM report dryly observes, "changed very little during 1983" (IOM 1995:76). And following the very public announcement that NIH in the person of Robert Gallo, had "discovered" the AIDS virus, "blood and plasma collection organizations, anticipating the quick development of a direct test for the virus, did not implement any additional donor screening procedures until such a test was developed" (IOM 1995:78). Once tests were developed, implementation of blood and donor testing turned out to be both complex and controversial. Beginning in late 1984 and for several years thereafter, the CDC

[39] Archived handwritten notes and memos point to a considerable gap between what informed members of the blood community admitted in private—i.e., AIDS is caused by a transmissible agent and is likely to spread—and what they were willing to acknowledge in public.

and the blood industry were consumed by the technical, social, and ethical dimensions of testing.[40] Perhaps seeking to bring some closure to this period, Curran reported to the U.S. Senate on June 24, 1987: "Eighteen months ago, among our primary concerns were ensuring the safety of our blood supplies and providing alternate testing sites for people who believed they may have been exposed to the AIDS virus. Since then safeguards have been put in place to make the blood supply safer; the alternate test sites have become counseling and testing programs; and AIDS health education/risk reduction programs are in place across the Nation" (U.S. Senate 1987:6. [Statement of James W. Curran]). Once blood and blood products were officially pronounced safe, threats to the blood supply and their ramifications disappeared—temporarily—from the federal agenda.

The Bark That Fell on Deaf Ears

The CDC was well positioned to declare a public health crisis in the early months of 1983. It had the data, dominated the scientific narrative of AIDS both among its peer agencies in the federal government and in public, and—unlike the French AIDS Working Group—it was an institutionally recognized player in the field of public health. Why, despite its best efforts, was the CDC unable to exploit this opportunity? And why—by comparison—did the pronouncements of a blood crisis in France over ten years later, when the blood supply was relatively safe, resonate so powerfully with political and public opinion? Here we address the first half of that question: Why did the CDC's alarm bells, grounded in the agency's expertise in both relevant biomedicine and epidemiology, go largely ignored?

The most obvious answer—and the one adopted by the IOM report—is scientific uncertainty: the absence of a clearly identified agent and AIDS's long incubation period that allowed a few cases to be readily dismissed as "rare" by CDC's interlocutors, while to the agency's trained investigators these cases were only the "tip of the iceberg." But as Michel Setbon observes, referring to a parallel reluctance on the part of French medical authorities at the same time (1983), "while scientific uncertainty is a partial explanation,

---

[40] The intensity, complexity, and controversy surrounding the implementation of blood testing are well documented in letters, memos, and reports deposited in James Curran's archives at the U.S. National Archives in Atlanta, Georgia.

it is insufficient to account for the total refusal . . . to see the possibility of an epidemic. To [admit that possibility] would be to disrupt an entire system" of long-established relationships and practices (Setbon 1993:59). The FDA's Bureau of Biologics, the blood industry, and the National Hemophilia Foundation together constituted just such a system (highlighted by Bruce Evatt in the interview cited earlier); their response to what they perceived as the threat posed by the CDC was to close ranks. *How* they perceived that threat is strongly suggested in a memo from Dr. Joseph Bove to the Committee on Transfusion Transmitted Diseases of the American Association of Blood Banks (AABB). Bove was simultaneously head of the AABB and of the FDA's Blood Products Advisory Committee (BPAC). The memo is dated January 24, 1983, two weeks after the Atlanta meeting. After stating that a recent case "increases the probability that AIDS may be spread by blood" and that "the most we can do in this situation is buy time," Bove goes on to say, "we do not want anything that we do now to be interpreted by society (*or by legal authorities*) as agreeing with the concept—as yet unproven—that AIDS can be spread by blood" (emphasis added). To acknowledge the threat of toxic blood was to anticipate massive legal liability. The strategies the CDC's rivals employed were (1) to impugn the CDC's historic record of success in tackling epidemics; (2) to undermine the CDC's scientific credibility; (3) to accuse it of "unscientific" (i.e., self-aggrandizing) motives; and (4) to call for blood industry solidarity.[41]

In January 1976 an army cadet at Fort Dix, New Jersey, died of a flu strain "closely related to the one that had caused the worldwide influenza pandemic in 1918 that had killed at least 20 million people" (Colgrove 2006:193). The CDC recommended mass vaccination of the U.S. population, multiple problems ensued including illness and and three deaths attributed to the vaccine, there was no flu epidemic, and the program was shut down three months after it began. The director of CDC at the time, David Sencer, was fired, and "the handling of the swine flu program was widely viewed as a debacle for all concerned" (Colgrove 2006:195). Presciently, the authors of a report on this incident commissioned by the U.S. Department of Health, Education, and Welfare observed that "if CDC should happen to foresee correctly the next public health disaster, then its loss of status may affect the lives of citizens"

[41] The term "rivals" is justified by the actions of the FDA in overruling the CDC's strong recommendations for protection of the blood supply and by the comments of blood industry executives presenting themselves in that light, e.g., "sticking together" against CDC, avoiding CDC to engage with NIH and the FDA instead, and the like.

(Neustadt and Fineberg 1978:98). Neustadt and Fineberg's prophecy was fulfilled, in spades. It is true—as in this case—that "actors consciously build on and/or react against previous governmental efforts for dealing with the same (or similar) problems" (Weir and Skocpol 1985:119), but actors also frame prior efforts in light of present interests and ideologies. The interests and ideologies of the CDC's rivals led them to make much of the swine flu "debacle" in order to discount the CDC's alarming reports.[42]

When speaking of scientific "uncertainty," it may be well to ask, whose uncertainty? Lack of scientific consensus is not the same thing as uncertainty. By the date of the Atlanta meeting, CDC scientists were certain that AIDS was caused by a viral agent transmissable through the blood supply to transfusion recipients and hemophiliacs. They simply were not believed. Comments cited earlier along with archived interviews and documents make two points: first, that credible "science" was perceived both within and outside the government (e.g., by the blood industry and also, perhaps, by journalists) as emanating from the NIH, not the CDC; and, second, that the CDC was seen by the FDA as encroaching on the latter's regulatory authority. Further—as even the IOM report acknowledged—BPAC had been captured by the blood industry long before the advent of AIDS. The CDC was framed by a chorus of rivals internal and external to the federal government as both a scientific and a bureaucratic upstart, allowing its claims to be dismissed.

Finally, the AIDS epidemic came along at the very beginning of the Reagan administration. As Curran remembers, "There was a hiring freeze at the CDC and a freeze on a lot of budgetary aspects of CDC, as well as a commitment to close the Public Health Service hospitals and to cut back on domestic spending. . . . So all this was going on in the background when the first [AIDS] cases were reported" (Curran 2/10/16 [CDC/Emory Collection]). It is in light of this same background, that the CDC's rivals portrayed the agency as "needing" an epidemic in order to justify its existence and going out of its way to court publicity. Despite these constraints, CDC as a collectivity of federal officials had both the scientific and organizational *capacity* to recognize the blood crisis and not only propose but also try to implement innovative strategies to contain it. What the CDC did not have—in contrast, for example, to the FDA—was the organizational *authority* and *autonomy* to

---

[42] Earlier predicted epidemics that did not materialize were also a factor in France's slow response to COVID-19 (Bergeron et al. 2020).

act independently of massive internal and external countervailing pressures (Carpenter 2010).

Gay Power

An additional argument advanced by the blood industry against CDC's proposals—specifically any form of donor screening that asked direct questions about sexual preference—was that it would be perceived as a form of discrimination: "The representatives of the gay groups point out in rather dramatic terms that during World War II we did some things to the Japanese people loyal to this country, that we now have a guilty conscience about—please let us not do the same thing to the gays" (BPAC 2/7/83). A second dimension of this argument was that gay men were excellent blood donors: "Relevant facts are: (1) the focal group of concern is the gays, we are not likely to incur much resistance with respect to elimination of any other group (i.e., Haitains and injection drug users); (2) as a proportion of the donor population only the gays are significantly greater than 1%; (3) homosexuals and bisexuals constitute up to 25% of the donor population" (American Red Cross internal memo, 2/5/83). These comments are from whole blood bankers and, as Healy (2006) has pointed out, this segment of the blood industry is organizationally highly dependent on its suppliers and loathe to antagonize them.

But the powerful impact of gay movement organizations on blood policy decisions in this early period of the AIDS epidemic in the United States had more complex origins and was more nuanced than Healy suggests. In sharp contrast with France, gay men's organizations—in particular gay physicians—had close ties with American health officials well before AIDS (Armstrong 2002, Curran interview, CDC/Emory Archives, February 2, 2016).[43] From the very first meetings on the blood supply convened by the CDC in the summer of 1982, physicians representing the National Gay Task Force and the Association of Physicians for Human Rights were invited, giving these groups a visible presence and legitimacy in blood policy deliberations.[44] The CDC and, in particular, James Curran and Donald Francis had a long history of working with gay physicians and with gay men more generally in the

---

[43] France had an association of gay doctors (Association de Médecins Gay [AMG]) whom Willy Rozenbaum contacted in the very early 1980s to provide information and bring them on board. Their initial reaction was quite hostile, but eventually a member of AMG joined the French Working Group.

[44] There was no such representation on FDA's BPAC.

course of STD surveillance and of ongoing research to develop a hepatitis B vaccine: "Well, [AIDS] was a new disease that affected a group [gay men] that [Dr. James W.] Jim Curran and I had considerable experience working with" (Francis interview, CDC/Emory Archives, October 13, 2016).[45] Given the larger political context of federal government indifference and stigmatization of a "gay" disease, the consistent presence of gay social movement representatives in the counsels of the PHS on AIDS/blood and the legitimacy they were accorded is striking.

Retrospective accounts by Curran and Francis make clear not only their close personal relationships with gay physicians but also their perception— one that contradicts much received wisdom on this topic—that the principal obstacle to more aggressive action to protect the blood supply was not gay men but the blood industry: "The gay community [in contrast to the blood banks], unlike the movie [*And the Band Played On*] presents them, was already (in January 1983) on board, and the major gay organizations were going along with the restriction of blood donations" (Curran interview, CDC/ Emory Archives, February 10, 2016). Curran's and Francis's perspectives may also reflect the CDC's commitment to protecting its cooperative relationship with gay organizations in light of an epidemic that in the early 1980s was still percieved as principally affecting gay men. The statement on AIDS published by the American Association of Physicians for Human Rights (AAPHR) in early 1983 and circulated in the gay press was more ambiguous than Curran's observation suggests. On the one hand, "individuals who think they might be at increased risk for AIDS should not donate blood"; on the other hand, "we object strongly to the attempts by some members of the blood products and blood banking community to identify gay men by questionnaire and exclude them from blood donation."[46] The AAPHR statement omits that the CDC had advocated for exclusion by questionnaire. This omission, we would argue, reinforces our emphasis on the complex network of relationships— both cooperative and antagonistic—that underlay early efforts at confronting the AIDS/blood threat in the United States, a level of complexity that raises

[45] The closeness of these relationships is poignantly reflected in an observation from Francis's oral history interview: "I stopped going to funerals in California because I knew so many people, really good friends of mine, who were really wonderful people in the AIDS community that did great things, that were now dying. I couldn't deal with it. There was so much death, and with this disease they're now my colleagues and friends that are dying" (Francis interview, CDC/Emory Archives, October 13, 2016).

[46] "Human Rights—A. I. D. S.," *Colorado Gay and Lesbian News*, April–May 1983, 11.

questions about simplistic explanatory accounts of this period grounded in "scientific uncertainty."[47]

French gays were no less incensed at the threat of "exclusion" from the community of blood donors than their American counterparts, but their response was fragmented. We commented earlier on the decline—even rejection—of political mobilization among gays in France during the early 1980s. While it would be a profound exaggeration to say that there was no homosexual community in France, it is fair to say that "there were no militant organizations that could be converted to the fight against AIDS" (Dulac 1992:63). Gay organizations did not want to talk about AIDS, AIDS organizations did not want to talk about gays, and French officials did not want to talk (at least not publicly) about homosexuals.[48] Dulac makes the interesting suggestion that one factor contributing to the relative political activism of American gays was the absence in the United States of a universal, dependable healthcare system, a gap that forced gays to create their own healthcare structures (and ultimately to provide the organizational clout that led to passage in 1990 of the Ryan White Act, ensuring there would be government-backed healthcare for people with AIDS). Differences in the structure and trajectory of social movement activism in the two countries are among the keys to understanding their patterns of response to toxic blood.

Hemophiliacs—the other "risk" group with a presence in the early U.S. meetings on AIDS—was represented by the NHF board chairman and members of its medical oversight committee (Medical Advisory and Scientific Committee [MASAC]). On January 14, 1983, less than two weeks after the Atlanta meeting on January 4, NHF convened its own "National Hemophilia Foundation/Industry Strategy" meeting. Those present included much the same cast of characters as at the Atlanta meeting, excluding gay organizations and the press. NHF's position on blood screening was much the same as that of the CDC—it wanted questionnaire-based exclusion of gay donors

[47] Based on subsequent research, Curran states that, in fact, "those [voluntary] blood donor restrictions did a great deal to protect the blood supply and saved thousands of lives, two years before the antibody test for HIV was available" (Curran interview, CDC/Emory Archives, February 10, 2016).

[48] This reluctance is strikingly illustrated by the first official French report on AIDS by Claude Got, published in 1989. The eloquent preface by then minister of health, Claude Evin, who requested the report, makes no reference to gays or homosexuals as special victims of this disease. Evin denounces demagogues who would exploit the epidemic for their own "moral" purposes and states "refusal of exclusion" as a principle of his proposed educational campaign against AIDS, but gays themselves are absent. Even more astonishing, they are absent from the report's chapter on "special problems," which includes headings for "mothers and children" and "drug addiction," but nothing on homosexuals.

and surrogate testing—and aligned with the commercial sector as well on the question of donor exclusion. The chairman of the NHF board "specifically pointed out that the medical rights of the Hemophiliacs transcended the civil rights of the gay community on this issue" (Cutter internal memo dated 1/17/83 [NAS Archives]). Nevertheless, at least for the time being, the preference of the gay community—and of the whole blood sector—for self-exclusion when it came to voluntary blood donation prevailed. Neither Haitians, injection drug users, or persons at risk of infection by transfusion were represented in these policy deliberations.

4

Act II—The Storm Breaks, 1986–1995

France

Recapitulation

Blood screening for HIV and heat treatment of blood products were introduced in France in 1985. The large majority of infections from HIV-contaminated blood happened in the years before those measures took effect. Most of the decisions later interpreted as scandalous—delay in authorizing the blood test and in heat treatment, failure to recall blood products known to be contaminated—were made in the spring of 1985 by those charged with responsibility for the blood supply, meeting behind closed doors. Their actions were unpublicized and invisible except within a very limited circle of blood and public health authorities.[1] There was no "crisis."

The Unraveling, 1986–1990

By 1987, the toll of sickness and death within the closed community of hemophiliacs had become visible to its members (Fillion 2009:145). The Association Française des Hémophiles (AFH, in English, French Association of Hemophiliacs) first approached officials of the Chirac government in the spring of 1987 to request help for families who had lost their bread-winner. There was no thought of accusation, merely "a gesture of solidarity for victims of technical progress" (Fillion 2009:145). A memo from the Direction Générale de la Santé (DGS) to the health cabinet dated January 14, 1988, argues that to comply with this request would create a bad precedent, implying assumption of responsibility by the state for hemophiliacs'

---

[1] Marchetti (2010) suggests that French journalists had been burned in 1983 by their aggressive treatment of an "affaire" involving hepatitis C vaccine made by Pasteur with imported American blood and were consequently restrained in their reporting of what they knew of events in 1985.

The Social Production of Crisis. Constance A. Nathanson and Henri Bergeron, Oxford University Press.
© Oxford University Press 2023. DOI: 10.1093/oso/9780197682487.003.0004

"infection with the AIDS virus"; transfusion centers are covered by insurance, and a preferable option would be for hemophiliacs to sue the centers individually. However, the memo goes on to state, if the state does get involved, there can be no question that it would have to cover the transfused as well as hemophiliacs (FNA, Box 910611-1 [CAB 506], January 14, 1988).[2]

On May 13, 1988, Claude Evin took office as minister of health in the newly elected Socialist government of Michel Rocard. Within a week of his arrival he received a letter from the Association de Défense des Polytransfusées (ADP, literally, Association of the Multiply Transfused). The ADP was organized in 1987 by dissidents from the Association Française des Hémophiles (AFH) to advocate publicly for the interests of hemophiliacs infected with HIV, in sharp contrast to the discrete strategy adopted by the AFH.[3] "The secret has been well guarded," read the letter to Evin. "You cannot know, but Madame Barzach [Evin's predecessor as minister of health] and Monsieur Chirac [prime minister in the previous government] knew the gravity of the situation. . . . The scandal has been deliberately smothered" (*Le secret a été bien gardé. Vous ne pouvez pas savoir, mais Madame Barzach et Monsieur Chirac connaissaient la gravité de la situation. . . . Il y a eu volonté délibérée d'étouffer le scandale*) (FNA: May 20, 1988).[4]

Health ministry cabinet documents from this period paint a complex portrait of officials driven by two projects inherently in conflict: (1) to craft a response to the repeated and increasingly importunate demands of organized hemophiliacs (both the AFH and the ADP); and (2) to keep the lid on a pot that constantly threatened to boil over, revealing the "unpublicized and invisible" actions of 1985 in a light now perceived as highly unflattering to their Socialist predecessors in power at that time (in 1985).[5] A memo to the Minister of Health from the cabinet member responsible for this issue (*dossier*, in French), dated March 30, 1989, and labeled "URGENT AND CONFIDENTIAL" (capitals in the original), gives some sense of the perceived

---

[2] All of the quotes from and references to cabinet documents in this chapter are from Box 910611-1, CAB 506, located in the French National Archives (FNA). Henceforth, we will abbreviate reference to those materials as "FNA" followed by the date.

[3] This association, organized by dissidents from the more traditional AFH will be fully described in Chapter 5.

[4] Unless stated otherwise, all letters, memos, and other documents cited were transcribed directly by Nathanson or Bergeron from the archived originals.

[5] The Socialist Party held the offices of president and prime minister from 1981 to 1993, except for the period, 1986–1988 (known as the *cohabitation*), when the National Assembly was taken over by conservatives and a conservative (Jacques Chirac) was appointed to the office of prime minister while the presidency continued unchanged (i.e., in the hands of Mitterrand).

threat: "This *dossier* is explosive and must be considered as a priority ... the individuals responsible for this issue (transfusion and health administration officials) know that it is explosive . . . . The solidarity of the different authorities predicated on silence is splintering now that the facts are gradually becoming known to the public and, in particular, to the victims" (*Ce dossier est explosif et doit être considéré comme prioritaire ... des gens qui ont géré ce dossier (responsables de la transfusion et responsables administratifs) savent qu'il est explosif. . . . La solidarité des différents responsables qui s'était réalisé autour du silence, éclate maintenant que les faits sont progressivement portés à la connaissance du public, et d'abord des victimes*) (FNA, March 30, 1989). It is evident from these documents that by early in 1989 (at the latest) members of the cabinet and of the Health Ministry's administrative services were fully cognizant of the actions taken in 1985; indeed, these actions had been spelled out in detail much earlier (August 1988) in a memo to a cabinet official from the president of AFH.[6]

As portrayed in these cabinet documents, breaking the silence that surrounded the interconnected events of blood contamination and infection of hemophiliacs was a gradual process, initiated by hemophiliacs but drawing in over the four-year period in question other actors, at first primarily journalists but eventually persons potentially implicated in these events, eager to defend themselves and point the finger elsewhere. Table 4.1 describes this trajectory.

The table begins in 1987 with the announcement of the formation of a group to represent the interests of the "multiply transfused" (the ADP) and ends in 1990 with the assertion by the French Association of Hemophiliacs (heretofore the government's "privileged interlocutor") that they, too, will go to court. All the entries in this table are from documents in the Evin cabinet archives, reflecting what cabinet members knew or believed at the time. Items in quotes are direct translations from cabinet memos or letters. Newspaper articles are included only if they were among the cabinet documents, meaning that they were read and filed by cabinet members.

Occurring simultaneously with the events documented in Table 4.1 were efforts by members of the Evin cabinet not only to address the demands of

---

[6] It is difficult to determine precisely who knew what when. In particular, given that the first detailed account of the events of 1985 (at least to our knowledge) is contained in this memo from AFH to the health ministry, it is plausible that AFH was the original source of information not only for the health ministry but for journalists as well. In an article published on April 26, 1989, in *Le Monde*, Garvanoff (the founder of ADP) is quoted as saying, "If the AFH knew all this, why didn't they say so?"

Table 4.1 Breaking the Silence

8/87	Notice of creation of the Association of the Multiply-Transfused hemophiliac victims of HIV contamination, to organize their interests and obtain compensation for the harms they suffered as the result of that contamination.
12/87	*l'Express*: "AIDS: The Tragedy of the Hemophiliacs."
2/88	*Le Monde*: "Many thousands of transfused are contaminated. . . . This situation, still little known to the public, appears to be particularly difficult for the government to manage."
6/88	"Media contacts indicate that Antenne 2 [TV channel] is preparing a broadcast on this issue [of contamination]."
10/88	*Agence France Presse*: "The Association of Hemophiliacs [AFH] calls on the government and public opinion to support 'measures of national solidarity' to benefit hemophiliacs infected by the AIDS virus."
1/89	"[This issue] is again going to be in the public eye. I [a cabinet official] am putting the brakes on [reporter for *Le Monde*] who has the whole dossier."
2/89	"[Reporter for *Le Monde*] announces the publication next Tuesday 22 February on the problem of contamination, with figures decidedly higher than those in our possession." "Mirko Grmek, in his *Histoire du Sida* [History of AIDS] . . . describes with precision the problem of transmission by blood transfusion." Best not to respond to television interview with Grmek, since a "partial justification . . . would only aggravate the polemics." "A large lobbying effort has developed directed at parliamentarians and the media."
3/89	"The solidarity of responsible authorities maintained around silence is splintering now that the facts are becoming public." "[Reporter for *Le Monde*] is playing on dissension among all those who want to pass the buck, and will come out with a new article in a few days." "The AFH holds its annual meeting the 29th and 30th of April and, confronted with pressure from victims, will break with the moderate approach it maintained heretofore. . . . Lawsuits will accelerate." "[Media] are acting as busybodies in this affair."
5/89	"The President [of AFH] is himself contaminated and only constant contact is preventing more spectacular actions. I [cabinet official] believe we will see a wave of lawsuits from ordinary transfusion recipients, which will increase the pressure."
8/89	AFH shares detailed account of 1985 events with *Le Monde*. Both the AFH account and the subsequent *Le Monde* article [August 26, 1989], titled "The Price of Errors," are in the cabinet archives. The article states that "up until now, only the Association of the Multiply-Transfused [i.e., not the AFH] has asked its members to bring criminal and civil suit."
11/89	"[Garretta] insists that the MOH take an official position on what happened in 1985 so that he himself is not the only one exposed. He implicitly threatens to implicate the Minister if he is not more fully supported." "I [cabinet official] think it best for the moment to have medical luminaries speak on this subject. I have asked [the chief administrator of public health services] to contact [elite French physician]." "Lawsuits in process threaten to amplify the debate."
2/90	"AFH . . . states that legal action by hemophiliacs is necessary since the compensation received so far is insufficient."

Note: All quotes and other notes are drawn from French National Archives Box 910611-1 (CAB 506).

hemophiliacs, as noted above, but also to construct alternative exculpatory and/or comforting narratives.

The State Is Not Responsible

The principal demand of the AFH was for financial aid from the state. The *principle* of aid in some form had been accepted by the health ministry under Barzach (i.e., early in 1988), in the hope (at least in part) of deflecting hemophiliacs from the pursuit of legal action.[7] However, under what label, from whom, with whose money, using what eligibility criteria, were matters of intense dispute, with the government insisting that it had no responsibility for the blood system, and hemophiliacs, along with executives of the blood system, insisting otherwise: "[The government's] strategy has always been to try not to be in the front line" (FNA, November 1989). Earlier in that year, this same official outlined the government's position more fully: "The central administration does not directly control the National Blood Transfusion Center (CNTS), much less the National Health Laboratory (LNS— Laboratoire Nationale de la Santé). The personnel of CNTS are not agents of the Administration and administrative responsibility cannot be invoked in this affair" (FNA, March 30, 1989). This position was maintained, at least officially, until 1992: the fund created by the government was labeled one of "solidarity," not compensation, framed to exclude any admission of fault (FNA, February 16, 1989). The AFH's dissatisfaction with this strategy is well documented: "The efforts of AFH between 1987 and 1989 to bring about a compensation fund came to nothing" (Fillion 2009:151). By contrast, the ministry official in charge of this dossier described himself as successfully staving off what he perceived as the excessive demands of AFH: "I stayed firm despite the blackmail of AFH (i.e., threats to join the ongoing legal action)" (FNA, February 22, 1990).

The Problem Was Not Preventable

A second narrative, bolstered by letters to *Le Monde* from celebrated medical authorities, was that HIV contamination of the blood supply and, hence, massive infection of hemophiliacs and transfusion recipients was

[7] Hermitte says Barzach encouraged hemophiliacs to bring suit against the blood centers, since they were insured for this purpose, and this assertion is consistent with cabinet documents cited earlier. AFH, however, was very reluctant to engage in legal action against these centers with whose personnel it had very close personal ties.

not preventable before the middle of 1985.[8] In correspondence between members of the cabinet and the health ministry's administrative arm, dated November 17, 1989, the latter notes that "controversy has arisen over the allocation of responsibility in 1985" and goes on to cite "medical experts" to the effect that that "these contaminations took place at a point when it was scientifically impossible to prevent them." This narrative is amplified (both in this correspondence and in other documents from the same period) with references to AFH support for blood system policies and policy decisions during 1985 and before.[9]

The Agitators Are Not Representative

Finally, the militants of the ADP were portrayed by cabinet officials as not representative of hemophiliacs: the new association of the multiply transfused "is trying to occupy the front of the stage; it has only a few members but has shown itself to be virulent and aggressive. . . . Hemophiliacs are largely represented by the [AFH], a partner well-known and respected by the government. The AFH should continue as the government's privileged interlocutor" (FNA, June 7, 1988). As late as November 1989, the ADP was being dismissed as a "very small but very active minority" (FNA, November 20, 1989).

"Not a Priority"

On the evidence from these documents and oral history interviews, hemophiliacs and contamination of the blood supply were not, despite the urgings of the cabinet member in charge of the dossier, a priority for the Evin cabinet. Reflecting on his experiences in that cabinet, an official with leadership responsibilities explained the cabinet was totally consumed with crafting a response to the larger challenge of AIDS: "The front page of *Le Monde* carried estimates of the number of potential AIDS victims in the years to come . . . [hemophiliacs and transfusion recipients] were just one

---

[8] This position was contrary to informed medical opinion outside of France, even at the time (see Chapter 3). On the evidence of the cabinet documents, at least one of these letters was actively solicited by representatives of the health ministry. The letter included with cabinet documents was signed by representatives of the blood system and by the president of the blood donor's association (but not by the AFH).

[9] There is ample documentation in the secondary literature and in newspaper accounts of AFH opposition (maintained up to and at least part way through the period 1988–1991) to any policies that would compromise the newly won autonomy of hemophiliacs gained through the use of easily injectable blood products (Hermitte 1996, Fillon 2009, Chauveau 2011).

more set of victims . . . not at all a priority" (Evin cabinet official, interview by author, November 4, 2010).

Cabinet archives from the period support this perspective. First, they document the intense preoccupation of Evin and his cabinet with development of prevention campaigns and construction of what would become in 1989 the Agence Française de Lutte Contre le Sida [AFLS—French Agency Against AIDS]. Second, contrary to the advice both of the DGS and of the cabinet, the press release stating that a fund supported by the government would be established for the assistance of hemophiliacs with AIDS was issued by the administrative arm of the Health Ministry, not by the minister himself, a clear indication to the actors involved of its minor importance in the hierarchy of political problems at the time.

Twenty years in retrospect, a key member of the Evin cabinet characterized this period as one of catastrophe, certainly not "scandal": "It [the blood affair] was not perceived as a scandal, not at all. It was a catastrophe. There were people who had been 'contaminated.'[10] That was how it seemed" (Evin cabinet official, interview by author, November 4, 2010). Using almost the same words, a recent book describes how "the drama of hemophiliacs 'contaminated' by the AIDS virus became, over a few months in the year 1991, the 'scandal of contaminated blood' " (Marchetti 2010:106). The story we tell is different. Constructing the "scandal of contaminated blood"—that is, reframing events from a "drama" of innocent victims into a "scandal" of preventable disease and government malfeasance—was a slow and highly contested process, the work of multiple actors with very different resources as well as goals and projects at stake. It was not until the spring of 1991 that the possibility of "scandal" crossed the boundary between hemophiliac "outsiders" and the state, compelling the latter into—at the very least—official engagement with the questions these "virulent and aggressive" outsiders had raised. Even that crossing did not happen overnight and was not fully accomplished until 1992, under the aegis of a new health minister appointed specifically for the purpose of coping with what at least some members of the government now identified as a "crisis."

---

[10] Note that in French discourse on this topic, both blood and people are "contaminated," not "infected," the somewhat more neutral word used in comparable English-language discourse.

Rupture, 1991

The impact of Casteret's "*j'accuse*," published on April 25, 1991, in a modest bi-weekly news magazine, buried in the back pages among full-page ads for cigarettes and mobile phones, bore all the classic earmarks of "crisis." It was experienced by the French public and elites alike as an "exogenous shock," a bolt from the blue. As described by a former cabinet official, "the revelation of scandal and not just catastrophe was certainly [Casteret's article] in *L'Événement du jeudi*. Before there were accusations, but it was her investigation that showed what really happened" (Evin cabinet official, interview by author, November 4, 2010). Practices well known to insiders and accommodated and accepted, even considered normative, by knowledgeable outsiders were suddenly made visible, held up to public scrutiny, and reframed as outrageous and appalling.[11] The article's author was a physician-turned-journalist, Anne-Marie Casteret, who had been following the blood story for several years and had in the late 1980s published other pieces on "the tragedy of the hemophiliacs." Reflecting with some bitterness on this article's profound impact on French society, Jean Yves Nau—journalist for *Le Monde* who with his colleague Frank Nouchi dominated medical reporting in France at the time of which we write (Marchetti 2010)—observed that "it wasn't her fault. It's the system that demands a Virgin Mary—a pure and innocent voice announcing catastrophe—a Don Quixote" (Nau, interview by author, November 4, 2011). Nau had, indeed, published several articles in *Le Monde* on the massive infection of hemophiliacs, including one precisely two years earlier (Nau 1989) that, in his own eyes at least, "contained all the elements of the '*dossier*' on the contamination of French hemophiliacs by the AIDS virus" (Nouchi and Nau 1991b). The essential difference between Casteret's article and French journalism on blood and death that had gone before was that while earlier articles (including her own) featured the victims—Nau's 1989 piece was headlined (in translation), "AIDS—The Scandal of Hemophiliacs," while Casteret's 1991 article centered on identified "perpetrators." In so doing, she attacked one of France's most sacred cows, its much beloved and admired blood system.

The extremely high levels of HIV infection and death among hemophiliacs were no secret to the Ministry of Health or, indeed, to any attentive reader

---

[11] We remind the reader that this conversion of known and accepted "contradictions" into outrageous normative departures is central to our conception of the social production of crisis.

of the French national newspapers. How, then, are we to interpret the virtually universal identification by scholars, politicians, and our interviewees of Casteret's article in 1991 as the "clap of thunder" that announced this scandal to the French public and ushered in a decade of tectonic shifts in the landscape of public health in France? What changed—as we will attempt to show—were not the facts of HIV infection but the meanings attributed to those facts. The "scandal" that Casteret revealed was not so much a health crisis as a cultural and political crisis, calling into question the legitimacy of one of the most revered institutions in France and implying a betrayal of the state's most sacred trust, to protect its population from disease and death. We begin this episode of our story with what Casteret actually said.

The centerpiece of Casteret's article—its provenance and allegedly incriminating language highlighted in large type—was a record of the meeting on May 29, 1985, of the executive committee of the Centre National de la Transfusion Sanguine (CNTS).[12] A copy of the document itself stamped "Confidential" was appended. The agenda for this meeting, stated in the minutes' heading, was "The attitude to adopt concerning HIV-positive blood donations discovered during [testing] and their incidence in blood products." The gist of Casteret's accusation was summarized in the article's subtitle: "In 1985, the CNTS knew that all of its concentrated blood products intended for hemophiliacs were contaminated with the AIDS virus. But these doctors continued to distribute them" (Casteret 1991:52).[13] Backing up these statements were direct quotes from the appended document: "With 2–3/1000 HIV positive donors . . . and lots of 1000 litres from 4–5000 donors, all our lots are contaminated" (Casteret 1991:52).[14] The most damning quote, however—its full import emerging gradually over the next few months—was CNTS director Michel Garretta's concluding statement that "it is up to the supervisory authorities (i.e., the State) to assume their responsibilities for this serious problem and possibly to prohibit us from distributing these products,

---

[12] Eight members of the committee were present at this meeting (two of whom were subsequently indicted, tried, and convicted). The doctors on the CNTS executive committee were among the elite of France's blood transfusion system and maintained close ties both with the French Association of Hemophiliacs and the Association of Blood Donors (e.g., as honorary members of their boards, members of their scientific committees, and the like).

[13] *"En 1985, le CNTS savait que ses concentrés destines aux hémophiles étaient tous contaminés par le virus du sida. Mais les médecins continuèrent à les distribuer."*

[14] It perhaps goes without saying that this conclusion was contested at the time and since. Nevertheless, even the sober government report requested by the Ministry of Health that appeared six months later and did everything possible to de-dramatize the blood affair, agreed that "lots" from the Paris region were undoubtedly contaminated.

with the financial consequences [that action] would represent" (Casteret 1991:52, emphasis added). In 1991 Casteret allowed those words to speak for themselves. In the 1992 introduction to her book, *L'Affaire du Sang,* she was more blunt: "The sick were coldly sacrificed to economic interests" (Casteret 1992:x). Her meaning had not been lost on *Le Monde* journalists Nau and Nouchi, however. In an article published on June 18, 1991, they link events in the month and a half since Casteret's publication (resignation of Garretta as director of the CNTS, launch of an official investigation, an escalating media-fueled search for guilty parties) to the "revelation" that transfusion doctors *had a financial interest* in their activities as physicians. We argued earlier that it was this revelation—the invasion of the market into the sacred domain of blood—that transformed the blood affair from *fatalité* to *scandale* and became the centerpiece of the dramas that were to follow.

It is critical to understand the full context of Casteret's "annunciation." Parallel to the unraveling of intragovernmental efforts to keep the blood affair under wraps was the simultaneous unraveling, first, of the extremely close—quasi-familial—ties among French hemophiliacs, their physicians, and the blood transfusion system and, second, of the internal solidarity among hemophiliacs themselves.[15] It is clear from the documents available to us—primary sources and the large secondary literature—that the facts recited by Casteret had been known to the French Association of Hemophiliacs since at least 1988 (and probably before), when the AFH's president transmitted a detailed recital of those facts to the minister of health (FNA, August 23, 1988). Nevertheless, much as the government worked to conceal the full extent of the blood affair, so the AFH—while threatening to make its knowledge public in pursuit of its demands for compensation—never did so. It was committed to working with the government as a privileged interlocutor—in contrast to more militant and litigious splinter groups—to devise a compensation strategy that would limit hemophiliacs' incentives to go to law. Above

---

[15] The intimate relationships between hemophiliacs, their physicians, and the blood transfusion system are described in detail in Emmanuelle Fillion's 2009 analysis of the French blood affair from the perspective of hemophiliacs, *À l'épreuve du sang contaminé: Pour une sociologie des affaires médicales.* "The ties between the population of hemophiliacs, totally dependent on blood products, and the transfusion system that monopolized their production were almost indestructible.... Annual meetings of the French association of hemophiliacs (AFH) were often occasions to see physicians, hemophiliacs and parents of hemophiliacs, blood donors—even local elected officials—celebrating the republican values of the French transfusion system" (134–35). From its founding in 1955, AFH headquarters was located on the premises of the CNTS in Paris. As was true of almost all French health voluntary associations prior to HIV, arbitration of medical and scientific questions was the undisputed domain of physicians.

all, the AFH was extremely reluctant to join lawsuits against the transfusion system: AFH representatives consistently maintained that responsibility for compensation belonged to the government, not the transfusion system. Cabinet documents and the work of Hermitte (1996), Fillion (2009), and Chauveau (2007, 2011) make clear both the increasing frustration of AFH representatives with its interlocutors within the government and the success of more militant hemophiliacs in putting the Association's feet to the fire.[16]

During the four years leading up to Casteret's article in 1991, the AFH confronted an increasingly splintered constituency, not only those hemophiliacs who organized independently to pursue a far more militant and litigious strategy but also dissidents within its own ranks: "At the core of the AFH, those who defended the preservation at all costs of relations with the physicians and the transfusion system found themselves more and more isolated" (Fillion 2009:155–56).[17] This tension is clearly reflected in cabinet documents of the period: "Tension is increasing enormously among hemophiliacs with the increase in sickness and death . . . the President of the AFH himself is infected . . . only constant contact [with the AFH] is preventing more spectacular actions" (FNA, May 30, 1989). By February of 1990, the AFH was "reluctantly" justifying legal action on the grounds that the sums hemophiliacs were receiving to date "were not nearly enough" (FNA, February 22, 1990).

Casteret's "thunderclap" was clearly a tipping point. But it was not quite the "clap of thunder in a cloudless sky of good health" portrayed by Grémy, nor was it a purely journalistic invention, as some others have suggested (see, e.g., Marchetti 2010). Both Hermitte and Fillion argue that the events of 1991 were prepared, first, by the emergence of militant collective action by hemophiliacs and, in particular, their initiation of legal action against the transfusion system, the AFH, and the government's National Scientific Laboratory (LNS) and, second, by their early collaboration with journalists to bring the "facts" to light: "[Hemophiliacs], convinced of having been poisoned, had convinced journalists that they had not only important information but the makings of a scandal. The journalists, in return, confirmed

---

[16] Members of the MOH cabinet met periodically with representatives of the AFH during the three years before the "explosion" in the spring of 1991 with the aim of devising a compensation strategy. From the hemophiliacs' perspective as documented by Fillion, "the efforts of AFH between 1987 and 1989 to bring about a compensation fund were unsuccessful" (*De 1987 à 1989, les démarches de l'AFH en vue d'une indemnisation n'aboutissent à rien.* [2009:151]).

[17] Some members of the AFH threatened to sue the AFH itself, a threat ultimately carried out by a leader of the most militant outside group (Hermitte 1996:349–50).

the conviction of the [hemophiliacs] by using the language of assassination, inhumane decisions, the interests of industry prevailing over those of health, and so on" (Hermitte 1996:350). The AFH shared office space with the CNTS. It does not require a great leap of imagination to speculate that the AFH itself was the source for Casteret's profoundly incriminating document. We turn now to the immediate (short-term) response to that article in major French newspapers[18] and to the actions of the principal actors implicated by Casteret: officials of the CNTS and government ministers.

A key element of the French response was clearly stated in the first article following Casteret to appear in Le Figaro, on May 30, 1991. "For the past two years, the AIDS-hemophilia drama has been a scandal in all Western countries. But in France this controversy takes a turn that is specifically 'hexagonal' [i.e., French]. The story of the deviations of the transfusion system . . . shows how a commercial and industrial strategy has put into moral bankruptcy a system founded on benevolence and nonprofit" (Strazzulla 1991a:7).[19] Hemophiliacs in the United States (starting rather later than in France) attacked pharmaceutical companies and the blood industry more generally for privileging its economic interests over public health (Bayer 1999). But the blood system in the United States had long been divided between nonprofit blood bank suppliers of whole blood and "commercial /industrial" suppliers of blood products relying on paid donors. There was never the illusion of an entire "system founded on benevolence and nonprofit" and no scandal was attached to making money from blood products.[20]

Le Monde, more hesitant than Le Figaro, waited until June 18 to state categorically that "some French leaders of the transfusion system had a financial interest in these activities" a fact that its reporters had no doubt would prolong a "virulent campaign" already in progress (Nau and Nouchi

---

[18] The two newspapers cited here are Le Figaro and Le Monde both national newspapers of record, published in Paris. Politically, the former is center-right, the latter center-left. It is important to remember, and we will return to this point, that the Socialist Party was in power both during the critical events of 1985 referred to by Casteret and in 1991, when her article appeared. Mitterrand, a Socialist, was president of France in both years.

[19] "Depuis deux ans, le drame hémophile-Sida fait scandale dans tous les pays occidentaux. Mais la polémique prend en France une tournure spécifiquement hexagonale. La chronologie de la dérive de la Transfusion française (dont les responsables assurent aujourd'hui n'avoir pas failli à leur mission) montre comment une stratégie industrielle et commerciale a mis en faillite morale un système fondé sur le bénévolat et le non-profit."

[20] The IOM report on "HIV and the Blood Supply," published in 1995, makes no mention of venality and greed as drivers of HIV infection in blood.

1991b).[21] In the meantime, on June 1 the most visible of those leaders, Michel Garretta, resigned his post as director of CNTS, claiming to be the victim of an orchestrated media campaign "of disinformation" with dramatic negative consequences for the blood system. On June 5, 1991, *Figaro* reported that criminal charges would be brought against Garretta along with the directors (in 1985) of, respectively, the DGS and the LNS, the two principal pillars of public health in France.[22] The French government's response, delayed until after Garretta's resignation (so over a month after Casteret's article first appeared), was, to say the least, incoherent. Within a period of three days between June 3 and June 5, the government's health ministers denounced the media for scaring off blood donors, stated on television that undoubtedly "serious errors of appreciation" had been committed, and requested an "objective, chronological" report from one of the government's watchdog agencies, the Inspector of Social Affairs (Inspection Générale des Affaires Sociales [IGAS]) (Strazzulla 1991c). Notably, the task of "objective" reporting was not given to a "scientific" committee (as it was—several years later—in the United States) but to the government. The initial reaction of the French medical elite to Casteret's exposé had been that she was "crazy," that what she described "could not have happened," that it was "impossible that these events were known and kept quiet" (Evin cabinet official, interview by author, November 4, 2010). These reactions may explain why elite physicians were not invited as disinterested observers. The Lucas report—named for its author, the inspector general of IGAS—was published in September 1991.

Finger pointing—the "questioning or discrediting of established policies, practices, and institutions" that is among the hallmarks of political crisis (Nohrstedt and Weible 2010:3)—had started before 1991 but was amplified and publicly reported in the months to follow. Interviewed by *Le Monde* on November 2, 1991, Bahman Habibi, Garretta's second in command at

[21] Several French writers have suggested that the principal reporters for *Le Monde*, Jean Yves Nau and Frank Nouchi, were close to Garretta (Fillion 2009:152), and, indeed, the first article in *Le Monde* to appear after Casteret (on the next day, April 26,) was a full-throated defense of Garretta. In later articles, Nau and Nouchi backed off of this defense but still occasionally referred to Garretta as a "*boucémissaire*" (scapegoat) and were active in enlarging the circle of wrongdoing to include more senior government officials. For *Figaro*, by contrast, Garretta was the devil incarnate.

[22] It is important to understand that the judge's decision was based on suits brought by hemophiliacs over the preceding three to four years, grounded in multiple legal theories. In this case, the hemophiliacs had the status of "third parties" (*parties civiles*). Their role is to convince the judge that their case crosses a certain legal threshold of harm. Once the judge decides to take the case, she then represents the "public interest" against the accused parties (see Hermitte 1996). It is plausible that the timing of the Paris judge's decision was influenced directly or indirectly by the media storm in progress, but this is pure speculation.

the CNTS (and among those present at the infamous meeting of May 29, 1985) commented about the fall-out from Casteret's revelations: "There followed an atmosphere destructive for everyone. It was the time for settling scores, between members of the CNTS, between people in the blood system, between the DGS and the ministerial cabinets, between the Socialist party and the Communist party, between different factions of the Socialist party, between the majority [socialist] and the opposition [conservative] and so on" (Nouchi 1991b). The drumbeat of media attention to what had become a front-page "scandal" continued through the summer and fall of 1991.[23] Purportedly incriminating documents were "newly discovered" by investigative journalists, including hitherto unpublished 1980 and 1985 reports by IGAS on the failures of the blood system. Events that had passed without comment when they occurred were resurrected by reporters and given new meaning: for example, under huge pressure from the French Association of Hemophiliacs, the government in 1989 in collaboration with insurers of the blood system had created a limited system of compensation conditioned on recipients' agreement not to sue either insurers or the transfusion system. On June 10, 1991, under the headline "How the Silence of the Contaminated Was 'Bought,'" the reporter described himself as "dumbfounded" by the "discovery" of a letter dated December 1989, titled "Private Fund Solidarity Transfusion—Hemophiliacs" informing the recipients of their eligibility for compensation and of the requirement that they refrain from suing (Nothias 1991a:36).

The myth of a blood system "removed from all questions of money" (Bruno Durieux, health minister at the time, quoted in Strazzulla, 1991b:13) was exploded not only by the evidence of CNTS involvement in blood commerce but also by the long drawn out battle—only finally resolved in 1992 under the aegis of a new health minister—over the amount, the conditions, and, above all, the meaning of compensation for those who acquired AIDS through whole blood transfusion or the injection of blood products. Fillion describes in fascinating—and, under the circumstances, poignant—detail the close, almost familial, relationships that had existed between hemophiliacs, their physicians (almost all of whom were women), and the local blood centers on whom hemophiliacs were dependent for the blood products that had by the middle of the twentieth century made it possible for persons (boys and

[23] Intense media attention to the blood affair did not begin until a month after the appearance of Casteret's article, coinciding with the resignation of Garretta.

men) afflicted with hemophilia to lead close to normal lives (Fillion 2009). The question of compensation—"the intrusion of money"—was perceived as incompatible with this domestic universe "based on connections of devotion and recognition which—by definition—had no price and constituted the uniqueness of the traditional transfusion clinic. . . . [And so this issue] created powerful tensions among patients, physicians, blood donors, and transfusion doctors: the traditional chain of solidarity around transfusion was broken" (Fillion 2009:153–54). Under enormous political pressure, a new and generous compensation package was endorsed by the government and passed by Parliament in December 1991.[24]

Among the most striking aspects of the immediate response to Casteret's revelations was the enormous solicitude of politicians (specifically government officials and members of parliament) for the bruised feelings of blood donors. The then minister of health, Bruno Durieux, chose the annual meeting of the French Federation of Voluntary Blood Donors (Fédération Française des Donneurs de Sang Bénévoles, FFDSB) as the forum for his first public comments following Casteret's publication (Strazzulla 1991b:13).[25] (This meeting took place at the Ministry itself, confirming the status of the FFDSB as a principal government interlocutor.) In an article headlined "Durieux Condemns the 'Polémique,'"[26] Durieux is quoted as praising the devotion to duty of blood transfusion leaders and personnel and asking donors to respond in kind (i.e., to continue and increase their donations) and to not be discouraged. At the end, the article reports, donors joined the minister in denouncing the "scandalous polémique" and expressing total confidence in "our blood doctors." Note that in this reading "scandal" has been redefined from its framing as an economically driven "contamination" of hemophiliacs to a media-driven attack on blood donors. In an interview given to Le Monde on June 7, Durieux reinforced this reading: "There are, on the one hand, hemophiliacs and transfusion recipients contaminated by the AIDS virus. There are, on the other hand, the consequences that a passionate treatment of this affair can provoke among blood donors. I mean that

[24] See Chapter 7.
[25] Durieux was not, in fact, a "full" minister of health but what is labeled a *"minister délégué,"* in other words subordinate in the ministerial hierarchy to the minister of social affairs, in this case Jean-Louis Bianco. Both Durieux and Bianco spoke for the government in response to the blood affair in 1991–1992, sometimes together, sometimes separately. Importantly, Durieux's successor, Bernard Kouchner, was a "full" minister.
[26] Google translates *"polémique"* as "controversy." "Controversy" lacks the emotive impact of "polemic," but polemic in English seems incorrect. Consequently, we have left the word in its original French.

the tone of certain articles risks demobilization and a profound loss of motivation among French blood donors. Blood donors today have the feeling of being attacked by what they perceive as a press campaign" (Nau and Nouchi 1991a). Concern that questions about the country's blood system might demobilize blood donors was by no means limited to French blood bankers (see, e.g., Healy 2006). But in the French case, this concern was rapidly overwhelmed by the mediatized drama of government misconduct.

By early September 1991, when the IGAS report "Blood Transfusion and AIDS in 1985: Chronology of Facts and Decisions Concerning Hemophiliacs" was published, the government's attention had moved from blood donors to its own survival. The same incriminating document published by Casteret was now released under the imprimatur of the government itself (along with thirty additional internal documents from the period) (Lucas 1991). Although the "press attack" on blood donors narrative never disappeared altogether, the Lucas report together with the criminal charges against Garretta and others made it increasingly difficult to sustain. Nevertheless, the ideological and organizational imperatives underlying Durieux's remarks cited above are important to understand. The French blood system was wholly dependent, certainly in principal and for the most part in practice, on donated blood (not only for whole blood, as in the United States, but for blood products as well). As Healy points out based on a comparison of the initial response to AIDS of "for-profit" and nonprofit blood suppliers in the United States, "an organization will move to protect the constituency it is externally dependent upon. Social-structural relations of relative power and dependency condition the interests of the organization, and valuable or important relations will be better attended to" (Healy 2006:96). For the French blood transfusion system, suppliers of blood—who had a choice whether to donate—were more important than recipients, who most of the time had little choice. And so (as we describe in Chapter 2) blood donation was sacralized and an entire organizational system—partaking of that sacralization—was constructed to ensure a relatively inexpensive and uninterrupted blood supply. It is little wonder that Durieux rushed to put his finger in the dike when the wall of sacralization threatened to crack.

Nau and Nouchi wrote in the fall of 1991 that one thing they could be certain of was that "the brutal discovery of a reality unknown to the public and poorly understood by physicians cannot but precipitate changes in an archaic system that [now] appears very different than the one—magnified and idealized because it was built on the benevolence of donors—to which we were accustomed" (Nau and Nouchi 1991c).[27] Embedded in these and other reporters' editorial comments and the commentaries these reporters elicited from public figures was a sense of betrayal on multiple levels: what we thought was pure—a Frenchman's blood—is now discovered to be dangerous; what we thought was sacred—a transfusion system built on republican solidarity—is now discovered to be profaned by the intrusion of filthy lucre; the medical profession whom we trusted is now discovered to have feet of clay; the government charged with protecting us has betrayed us. By November 3, 1991, the once and future conservative health minister and prominent public figure, Simone Veil, was on television stating that public health in France was a "failure" (Nau and Nouchi 1991d).

Amplification, 1992

Once launched, the blood crisis took on a life of its own. The elements of its amplification in the public sphere included expansion in the range of institutions involved as accusers or accused (or both), in the number and political prominence of persons accused, in the gravity of their alleged wrongdoing, and in the sheer volume of journalistic and literary attention. As Poumadière and Mays observed about a spate of unexplained fires in the south of France: "Responses to the risk event [here the allegations in Casteret's article] actually define the risk itself: the construction of the event . . . shared in interaction and in collective sense making, itself shapes the danger" (2003:209). As the (retrospectively identified) danger became increasingly politicized, its perceived seriousness and the force of demands for retribution and repair increased correspondingly. Although there were multiple actors in this drama, the most vocal—those who had the ear of journalists and to whom journalists went for new angles on the blood story— were self-identified "victims," militant and litigious hemophiliacs and, later, persons who acquired HIV through transfusion. Physicians who treated hemophiliacs were both angry at their seemingly ungrateful patients and largely silent (see, e.g., Fillion 2009:57–58) as was the normally loud voice of organized blood donors.

---

[27] "on ne dispose aujourd'hui que d'une certitude: la découverte brutale d'une réalité infectieuse jusqu'ici ignorée du grand public ou trop mal connue du corps médical ne peut que précipiter l'évolution d'un système archaïque qui, jour après jour, apparaît bien différent de celui _ magnifié et idéalisé parce que bâti sur le bénévolat des donneurs _ que l'on avait coutume de présenter » (Nau and Nouchi 1991c).

The Lucas report was quickly followed in the fall of 1991 by the appointment of a Commission of Inquiry by the French Senate. Hearings before this Commission as well as the trial of blood bankers and government officials indicted in the spring of 1991 continued well into 1992. The Senate's report, published in the spring of 1992, was harsh in its indictment of a blood system led astray by overweening ambition and economic greed. The trial covered by the media in excruciating detail—"it was headline news for four months"—dwelt on much the same themes. It was accompanied by protests organized by Act Up-Paris. Cries of "AIDS—The politicians knew—They murdered" resounded through the open windows of a crowded and sweltering courtroom. Act Up's language accurately reflected both militant victims' belief that the officials brought to trial were scapegoats for the high-ranking ministers and their cabinets who were truly at fault and that the product liability theory under which the two blood bankers and their two nominal superiors had been brought to trial was totally inadequate to what the victims framed as murder.

Accusations that ministers were directly responsible for blood contamination increased exponentially during 1991 and 1992, nurtured by well-publicized gaffes in the public statements of ministers and by a conscious effort on the part of some journalists to take the blood story beyond a tale of innocent victims to one of ministerial and political responsibility (interview, Nau 2010). Georgina Dufoix, health minister in 1985 during the key period of decision-making on measures to ensure safety of the blood supply, famously described herself as "*responsable mais non coupable*"—responsible but not guilty—bringing down the wrath of hemophiliacs and precipitating opposition political parties to demand that charges be brought "at the highest political level" (*Le Monde*, November 5, 1991, cited in Steffen 1999:96). On April 11, 1992, in what was described by one of our informants, a former cabinet official, as a "bomb" dominating the press for weeks afterward, *Le Monde* on its front page published the first of two articles on blood collection in prisons headlined: "The High Proportion of Persons Infected in France Following a Blood Transfusion Is Explained in Part by Blood Collection in Prisons" (Nau and Nouchi 1992). These journalists cited "unpublished" documents purporting to demonstrate the extreme reluctance of public officials to act in the face of prisoners' demonstrably high rates of drug use, hepatitis, and AIDS known, according to Nau and Nouchi, as early as 1983. Reluctance to end this high-risk activity was attributed not only to its ease and low cost in the face of high demand but also to its importance for prisoners' rehabilitation. At a meeting of the *Commission Consultative de Transfusion Sanguine* (CCTS) toward the end of 1985, the head of one of France's largest blood banks expressed his concern that preventing detainees from giving blood would lead to feelings of isolation and the loss of an argument for early parole based on the good character demonstrated by blood donation (FNA, November 11, 1985). But Nau and Nouchi's point was not so much to debunk French blood mythology, as to enlarge the scope of responsibility for blood contamination: "One cannot, any more than with hemophiliacs, limit oneself to demonizing a tiny number of authorities who maneuvered diabolically for monetary gain to poison sick people" (Nau and Nouchi 1992).

The potential culpability of ministers in office in 1985—including the prime minister—had been suggested in reports by the Senate and the National Assembly and in the original indictment of blood banking officials in 1991. In the summer of 1992, hemophiliacs petitioned the Senate and the Assembly demanding that ministers be indicted. That fall, the two conservative parties in Parliament passed resolutions supporting this position. The Socialist majority demurred on the grounds that the French Constitution did not allow for the indictment of ministers. President Mitterrand, however, took the position that ministers should be allowed to defend themselves at trial and called for a constitutional amendment to that effect. The necessary amendment was passed in 1994 after a 1993 change in government that brought the conservatives to power. Under this new constitutional regime, some thirty people were indicted under various legal theories, including poisoning and involuntary homicide. Following nearly ten years of legal maneuvers, the bulk of these accusations were dismissed in 2003 on the grounds of "no proof that [the defendants] intended to harm people or that they even knew that the blood stocks were contaminated" (Casassus 2003:2019).

The blood crisis led to immediate and substantial institutional change in the field of public health in France (Bergeron and Nathanson 2012, Nathanson and Bergeron 2017).[28] Public health itself was reinvented as "*sécurité sanitaire*," a far more socially and historically resonant conception of the state's responsibility for disease prevention as well as medical care. New state institutions to manage the blood system, to regulate pharmaceuticals (now expanded to include blood products), and to conduct disease surveillance suddenly came into being. The power of elite physicians waned (at least temporarily), and the voices of newly organized patients were heard at

---

[28] We describe these changes in more detail in Chapter 10.

hierarchical levels where they had previously been invisible. We will return to questions about the relation between crisis and change in the book's final chapter. We turn now to what was happening in the United States during the period of acute crisis in France.

United States

"Hiding in Plain Sight"[29]

By 1985, when the blood supply had become relatively secure, 75% to 85% of American hemophiliacs—some 8,000–10,000 people—were HIV positive (Korner et al. 1994). Among transfusion recipients, approximately 29,000 were infected (Bayer 1999:34). *And the Band Played On*, Randy Shilts's path-breaking tale of the early years of the AIDS epidemic, was published in 1987. Artfully worked into Shilts's 621-page "medical sleuth story" was a detailed account, based on his reporting and interviews, of how the blood supply had become contaminated in the United States and France. Shilts's focus in this narrative was not on "irresponsible" blood donors (as the focus came to be later under the influence of Senator Jesse Helms and others) but on the extreme reluctance of blood bankers to recognize the threat of AIDS to the blood supply and to take steps to mitigate that threat. Reviews in the mainstream press barely mentioned this side of the story. It was buried, not deliberately perhaps, but lost in the flashier story of AIDS, gays, and "patient zero." Although Shilts had made the massive HIV infection of hemophiliacs quite clear, we were unable to locate a single review, in mainstream or local press, in *Science* or *Scientific American*, or in academic journals that mentioned this fact.

In September of 1989, Gilbert Gaul, an investigative reporter for the *Philadelphia Inquirer*, wrote a series of Pulitzer Prize–winning articles on the blood industry in the United States as devastating in its portrayal of blood bankers' privileging of profit over safety and of government regulatory neglect as anything published in France. Douglas Starr in his comprehensive history of the blood industry states that "Gaul's revelations scandalized the

---

[29] When asked about sources for his 1989 articles on the blood supply in the *Philadelphia Inquirer*, Gilbert Gaul described hemophiliacs as "hiding in plain sight" (personal communication 2021).

[American] public" (1998:260). In a careful review of news coverage at the time, we were unable to find any evidence of public scandal. On the contrary, among the consequences of Gaul's articles was to shut down significant coverage of the blood story in other major newspapers—"other papers conceded the ground to us" (Gaul, personal communication, 2021).[30]

The *Inquirer's* series did, however, trigger congressional hearings on blood safety. Under the chairmanship of John Dingell (D-MI), the House Subcommittee on Oversight and Investigations of the House Commerce and Energy Committee had a fourteen-year history of scrutinizing the actions of federal agencies, including the FDA. According to journalist Judith Reitman, "the blood scandal among the nation's 20,000 hemophiliacs" had caught the attention of Dingell's staff director, "but the hemophiliac community was a relatively small one. *It didn't have the kind of national scope [the staff director] needed to put before a Dingell subcommittee*" (1996:85, emphasis added). He found the scope—and drama—he was seeking in Gaul's depiction of the American Red Cross as the highly secretive leader of a multibillion-dollar blood industry.[31] The intent of those hearings on "Blood Supply Safety" was stated unambiguously in Dingell's opening statement on July 13, 1990:

> This inquiry has its roots in the early to mid-1980's when the blood industry and the Government failed to prevent transfusion of thousands of pints of blood and blood products infected with the AIDS virus. Today, however, *our focus is on the present and not on the past*, and this investigation will be directed towards answering the question of whether the blood supply is as safe as it could be or as it should be and to also ascertain what it is that we should do to assure that the best possible steps are taken to assure safety of all persons involved in this very important human activity. (U.S. House of Representatives 1990, emphasis added)[32]

Dingell was fully aware, of course, of what his first four witnesses were going to say. Apart from their prepared statements for the Subcommittee, two were prominent and outspoken AIDS experts who had been extensively

---

[30] Gaul's explanation was that the competitive posture of major national newspapers at the time caused them to ignore stories that another paper had taken up. For example (as recounted by Gaul), the *Wall Street Journal* had itself been about to break an investigative report on the blood industry but killed it when the *Inquirer's* story was published (Gaul, personal communication, 2021).

[31] In personal conversation, Gaul confirmed Reitman's story and his ongoing communication with Dingell's staff as they laid the groundwork for the blood safety hearings.

[32] We also refer to the series of hearings held by this subcommittee as the "Dingell hearings."

quoted by Shilts. In language that bore a marked resemblance to the French Senate report two years later, they told the Subcommittee that clear and authoritative warnings of an HIV-contaminated blood supply were ignored by blood bankers and by the FDA; that these warnings dated from 1983 at the latest; and that there was "collusion" among the three principal American blood banking groups to play down the threat, prompted by financial considerations. Nevertheless, Dingell had made it clear that raking over this history would not be part of his committee's brief. It was largely ignored in subsequent hearings before Dingell's committee and in those hearings' scant media coverage. Dingell's committee rapidly narrowed its focus to ongoing problems in the American Red Cross's blood program. In the course of four hearings in 1990, 1991, and 1993, irregularities that occurred before 1985 were treated as old history; members stated repeatedly that the hearings should avoid creating public "panic" about the blood supply's safety; and one member congratulated his colleagues that any problems in the United States were not as bad as the French, "where governmental officials deliberately released contaminated blood into the blood supply" (U.S. House of Representatives 1993:18). Nonetheless, these public hearings and the documents they brought to light were critical to the growing recognition among a minority of American hemophiliacs of the processes that led to their massive HIV infection (oral history interview, Resnik Archives, September 9, 1991).[33] It was early in 1993 that they first approached members of Congress to demand a full-scale investigation of the "old history" that transpired in the early 1980s.

One month before the start of the Dingell hearings, Senator Jesse Helms (R-NC) used the first day of Senate debate on the Ryan White Care Act to describe the young hemophiliac in whose honor this legislation was named as "an innocent victim of these people" making quite clear that by "these people" he meant gays and injection drug users (Cong. Rec., May 14, 1990).[34] Helms went on to attack the "AIDS propaganda machine [that] churned out the demand for special treatment and privileges for the kind of people who caused Ryan White's death" (Cong. Rec., May 14, 1990). The Care Act was

---

[33] Dana Kuhn, the author of this interview, was a hemophiliac with HIV and an early spokesperson and advocate on behalf of HIV-infected hemophiliacs in the United States.

[34] All direct quotations in this paragraph are drawn from floor debate on the Ryan White Act (S2240) as reported in the *Congressional Record*. The full citation is Congressional Record, 101st Congress (1989–90), https://www.congress.gov/bound-congressional-record/1990/05/14. We have simplified the in-text citation to Cong. Rec. plus the date.

framed by its sponsors as disaster relief, an indispensable infusion of federal funds to support the medical care of multiplying numbers of persons with AIDS. A few days after his first intervention, Senator Helms proposed an amendment to the Care Act making it a federal crime punishable by fine or imprisonment or both for an individual who was HIV infected or an injection drug user or a person engaged in prostitution to donate or attempt to donate blood. Helms described his amendment as intended to "ensure the safety of the blood supply of this Nation" by "[giving] pause to some of these people who have done, and might do again, this dastardly act of providing the kind of blood that caused the death of little Ryan White" (Cong. Rec., May 16, 1990). Sponsors of the Care Act (Senators Edward Kennedy [D-MA] and Orrin Hatch [R-UT]) deflected this amendment, not by opposing the principle of criminal responsibility for knowingly donating bad blood but by kicking the can to the states. The Kennedy-Hatch alternative amendment precluded states from receiving funds under the Care Act unless "the Secretary of Health and Human Services . . . determines that the criminal laws of that State are adequate to prosecute any individual who knowingly and intentionally donates or attempts to donate blood if the person has been diagnosed to have the HIV virus, and has been informed that he or she is infected and has knowledge of the risk of transmission of such virus through the donation of blood, blood products, semen, tissues, organs, or other bodily fluids" (Cong. Rec., May 16, 1990). The Helms amendment was defeated by a vote of forty-seven in favor fifty-two opposed, on entirely partisan lines. Not a single Republican voted against an amendment with the singular purpose of criminalizing selected blood donors, and no Democrat voted for it. The Kennedy-Hatch substitute amendment went on to pass almost unanimously. In the course of debate, Senator Kennedy cited opposition to the Helms amendment from the American Red Cross, the American Association of Blood Banks, and the National Hemophilia Foundation; letters from these organizations were inserted in the hearing record.

Senator Jesse Helms converted Ryan White into a symbol not just of "innocent" AIDS victims but also of the threat to the blood supply represented (in his narrative) by gays and drug users.[35] In so doing he effectively politicized the question of blood safety, making it extremely difficult for Democrats to embrace the cause of hemophiliacs without alienating gay organizations

---

[35] It is clear from Helms's references to "lobbying" and the "AIDS propaganda machine" that gays were the principal target of his amendment.

at the same time. Gay leaders were fully aware of their community's political vulnerability. Bayer cites an article in the *New York Native* from August 1982, shortly after the first CDC report of three cases of AIDS in hemophiliacs, warning "against a return to the bad old days . . . when a recurrently scapegoated minority could be sweepingly restigmatized for the taint of bad blood" (1999:22). In 1983, the National Hemophilia Foundation was denounced by "the National Gay Task Force and more than 50 other gay political, social, and medical organizations" for its position demanding the exclusion from blood donation of gay men and other high-risk populations (Bayer 1999:22). Not only was the gay community an important Democratic Party constituency, also a key partner in the fight against AIDS. Blood bankers—the American Red Cross, the American Association of Blood Banks, and others—had positioned themselves as opposed to the "exclusion" of gay blood donors and as strong supporters of the Ryan White Care Act. Given these organizational and political dependencies, it is perhaps no wonder that staunch Democrat John Dingell preferred to consign "mistakes" made in the 1980s to a distant past and that (as we shall see) a Democratic administration was markedly lukewarm to hemophiliacs' quest for compensation driven by conservative Republicans.

It was not only Democrats that shied away from a direct attack on blood bankers.[36] In floor debate on the Helms's amendment the possibility of criminal behavior by the bankers and industrialists who *processed* blood was never mentioned. Only individual *suppliers* were potentially at fault. This is the mirror image of what happened in France, where efforts at criminalization were focused entirely on processors, never on donors.

Blood Brothers

Among the most intriguing subplots in the American blood story is the equivocal role of the FDA. Beginning in the late 1980s the Agency's "failure" to carry out its responsibility for protection of the blood supply at a moment when this supply was uniquely at risk was denounced in multiple public forums. Earlier, we quoted the rather bland observation from the IOM Committee to Study HIV Transmission Through Blood and Blood Products

---

[36] Dingell was not at all hesitant going after *current* misbehavior of the Red Cross. He was powerfully averse to dredging up the past.

that "the agency [the FDA] did not adequately use its regulatory authority and therefore missed opportunities to protect the public health" (IOM 1995:7). Others were more blunt. Gaul's front-page story in the *Philadelphia Inquirer* on September 25,1989, read: "The Loose Way the FDA Regulates Blood Industry." Testifying before the Dingell Committee in July 1990, Marcus Conant, a professor at the University of California Medical Center and founder of the San Francisco AIDS Foundation, stated, "the blood industry failed us, the CDC failed us and finally the FDA failed us. The regulatory Agency charged with overseeing the blood banking industry published recommendations that at best were nothing more than watered-down recommendations from the blood banking industry itself" (U.S. House of Representatives 1990:11).

In a later hearing of the same committee, David Kessler, newly appointed as FDA commissioner in 1990, described the FDA's relationship with the blood industry "at that time" (i.e., in the early 1980s):

> [Blood banking] grew up . . . as a cottage industry [and] it developed almost a cottage industry mindset. . . . No one realized . . . that what was really going on was that they were manufacturing a product. . . . Some companies still see FDA regulation as a paper game. They establish an operating procedure on paper because they have to do it, but they don't bother to follow it up . . . blood banks have had to make a shift to see themselves as a regulated industry. . . . This has also required a shift for FDA and particularly for our Center for Biologics Evaluation and Research, known as CBER. . . . [Past FDA actions were] emblematic of our collegial approach to a regulated industry. . . . Those days are behind us. We have shifted, from relying on voluntary agreements to the use of agreements involving court supervision and sanctions where necessary, from concentrating on jaw boning with industry to writing enforceable regulations. Today, there is not a reluctance on the part of the Agency to take strong action when necessary." (U.S. House of Representatives 1993)

The implication of Kessler's testimony is that prior to his assumption of FDA leadership, the blood industry—in contrast to "other regulated industries"—was a law unto itself heeding the FDA, or not, as it saw fit. Accusations against the FDA were loudly echoed in the testimony of hemophiliac representatives before the IOM committee and by members of Congress in support of compensation for hemophiliacs who had died of AIDS and their families.

Nevertheless, not only was there no official investigation—and certainly no prosecution—of the FDA arising from its alleged failures, but also—and even more remarkable in our view—major recent scholarly works on the FDA make no reference to the blood story.

Perhaps the most persuasive explanation of these omissions comes from the most eminent of those scholars, Daniel Carpenter. Recognizing that despite its wide acclaim, the FDA "was just as often assailed as praised." Carpenter argues that, paradoxically, "the Administration's reputation persisted because of the acrimony itself. The ceaseless contestation of the organization's power and its image yielded not an abiding uncertainty about the Administration, but instead a persistence of the metaphors representing it. . . . Every criticism embedded a portrait. And every portrait displayed an organizational capacity that someone in the pluralistic soup of American national policy could admire" (2010:301).[37] Eyal suggests two hypotheses to account for the FDA's imperviousness. First, "the reputation of the regulator and the credibility of its scientific methods have become an integral part of the product the pharmaceuticals are selling" (2019:133). Damage to the reputation of the FDA would rebound on consumer trust in the product and expose manufacturers to legal liability. Second (and more important from our perspective) the actions of the FDA take place within "networked congeries of audiences—[pharmaceuticals,] pivotal professional and scientific networks, consumer representatives, media organizations" and the staff of the FDA itself. "Every attack on the FDA, every condemnation, inevitably also reactivated [symbolic reputational beliefs] thereby mobilizing a counter-audience invested in them" (Eyal 2019:135).

Internal correspondence immediately following the 1983 CDC meeting make clear not only the rapid mobilization of both the manufacturing and the blood-banking arms of the industry in the face of what they perceived as financial and potential legal threats to their business but also their solidarity with the FDA.[38] In a memo dated January 17, 1983, reporting on a meeting of "the major [pharmaceutical] industry representatives . . . to determine a consensus strategy," the reporter wrote: "We . . . agreed that the CDC was getting

[37] One need go no further than Congressman John Dingell himself, among the FDA's severest critics, to illustrate Carpenter's point: "America can look to its food, America can look to its cosmetics, America can look to its appliances, to its blood and every other commodity that affects health and that sustains life and know that it is safe because of the Food and Drug Administration" (quoted in Kessler 2001:317). Note that Dingell made this statement in 1996, well *after* the close of his hearings on the blood affair. Testimony about FDA "failure" had little impact.
[38] See Chapter 3 on the CDC meeting.

increasingly involved in areas beyond their area of expertise and whenever possible we would try to deflect activity to the NIH/FDA. Apparently there were some major differences of opinion voiced at the ABRA [manufacturers' association] meeting last week between Evatt [CDC] and Donahue [FDA]." A week later, Joseph Bove, the head of the FDA's Blood Products Advisory Committee (himself a blood bank director and officer of the American Association of Blood Banks [AABB]) wrote to his AABB colleagues, "The difficulty was to get AABB, ARC, CCBC and all the other groups to adopt a position which was acceptable to each other. . . . We have had a good start at working together on this, and we want to keep it up. . . . I hope we are equipped psychologically to continue to act together. We plan frequent conference calls to keep each other informed . . . we were helped by participants from the National Gay Task Force" (IOM 1995, Appendix D:281).

In an almost perfect illustration of Eyal's hypotheses, the FDA's networked audiences mobilized to protect themselves—and the FDA itself—against the loss of trust and legal liability threatened by HIV contamination of the blood supply and against the CDC that carried the bad news. This is in sharp contrast to French blood bankers who (as noted earlier) rapidly splintered once the discovery of HIV in the blood supply and its implications were made public in 1991.

We turn now to more detailed accounts of hemophiliacs' emergence as a political force in France and, later, in the United States, of militant hemophiliacs' struggles to obtain redress through litigation and/or financial compensation by the state, and of how various parties (courts, official commissions, political bodies, the press, academics) in the two countries framed what was "known" about HIV in the blood supply, when it was known, the limits and validity of that knowledge, and who (if anyone) among the multiple actors in this drama was "responsible"—for knowing and for acting on that knowledge.

5

Mobilization of the Afflicted

In the summer of 1993, Jean Peron Garvanoff was dying of AIDS. Every day when the court was in session, he drove fifty miles from his home outside of Paris to attend the appeal against their sentence of the officials convicted in 1992 of fraud in the merchandising of blood products, occasionally shouting "Assassin!" when outraged by arguments for the defense (Kramer 1993). Little more than a year later, hemophiliacs, their spouses, and children crowded into the ornate halls of the Institute of Medicine (IOM) in Washington, D.C. to give oral testimony to their lived experience of suffering and betrayal before the IOM "Committee to Study HIV Transmission Through Blood and Blood Products." Persons—boys and men—with hemophilia, their parents, and their wives were galvanized into collective action by the cascade of deaths among their brothers, spouses, and children. Neither in France nor in the United States did hemophiliacs engage in public protest on the scale of gay men. Nevertheless, without contentious action on the part of organized hemophiliacs and their allies, there is very little likelihood that either government would have acted to provide some level of compensation[1] and even, perhaps, to reform their countries' blood systems, certainly not in the United States and possibly not in France. The critical importance in the United States of pressure from an organized grassroots movement is reflected in the fact that individuals infected through whole blood transfusion were not compensated despite some obvious parallels with hemophiliacs.

The worlds of French and American hemophiliacs in the 1970s and early 1980s before the shattering intrusion of AIDS were remarkably alike. The disease itself often entailed a life-long and sometimes intense relationship between doctor and patient in the context of settings that brought parents and their sons, adult hemophiliacs and their wives, and treating physicians and nurses together, creating small, relatively insulated, and highly particular

---

[1] Officials in both countries pushed back against the word "compensation" (*indemnisation* in French) as implying government responsibility for fault.

The Social Production of Crisis. Constance A. Nathanson and Henri Bergeron, Oxford University Press.
© Oxford University Press 2023. DOI: 10.1093/oso/9780197682487.003.0005

communities (Fillion 2009, Resnik 1999).[2] Both countries had associations of hemophiliacs well positioned—at least in theory—to warn their members in the early 1980s about the newly discovered dangers of blood products and to advocate for those who were stricken by AIDS. Each of those associations— the Association Française des Hémophiles (AFH) and, in the United States, the National Hemophilia Foundation (NHF)—were embedded in a dense field of overlapping relationships with treaters (physicians and nurses), blood bankers, experts in the fields of hematology and transfusion, manufacturers and distributors of blood products, and government regulators. Makers of blood products—CNTS (Centre National de Transfusion Sanguine) in France and pharmaceutical companies in the United States—supported these associations financially, including space for the French association's offices in Paris; outside of Paris the association located its offices on the premises of regional transfusion centers. And in both countries these traditional— and relatively conservative—associations came to be regarded with suspicion by some HIV-positive hemophiliacs who split off and formed their own more militant groups. Among militants' principal accusations was their associations' failure to warn of the risk of AIDS from injecting contaminated blood products—a risk of which they maintained these associations, or at least their medical committees, were fully aware. Indeed, until late in 1985 both the AFH and the NHF minimized the risk of AIDS, assimilating it to the risk of hepatitis, a serious side effect of blood therapy and long regarded as an acceptable trade-off for the benefits of biotechnological innovation (IOM 1995, Carricaburu 2000, Fillion 2009). From the perspective of both hemophiliacs and the physicians who treated them, those benefits were huge, allowing the former to lead a relatively ordinary life free from the constant threat of hemorrhage and hospitalization while enabling the latter to effectively "cure" patients who before the advent of an easily administered blood-clotting factor had been doomed to constant medical oversight and early death.[3] Beginning in 1983 and through 1985, French blood experts

---

[2] Keshavjee, Weiser, and Kleinman (2001) state that hemophiliacs and their families in the United States only became a community as an outcome of the AIDS tragedy. Resnik (1999) makes clear that their common experience with the disease in treatment centers and other venues brought many of them—not all—together much earlier.

[3] The impact of Factor VIII (AHF) on the lives of hemophiliacs was at least equivalent to the impact of anti-retrovirals on the lives of persons with or at risk of HIV and comparable to—if substantially greater than—the impact of vaccines for COVID-19. It is not difficult to imagine the consequences if PrEP was suddenly discovered to be lethal. Current vaccine hesitancy in France has been attributed to the continuing ripples of the blood affair (*Science*, "Vaccine-Wary France Turns to Citizens' Panel to Boost Trust in COVID-19 Shots," February 18, 2021).

alternated warnings—hemophiliacs should shift to safer, if less convenient, blood-clotting measures—with reassurance—the risk of AIDS was much less than that of hepatitis. In the United States, the NHF, responding in May 1983 to a manufacturer's recall of AIDS-contaminated concentrate, urged "that patients and treaters recognize the need for careful evaluation of blood products and that such a recall action *should not cause anxiety or changes in treatment programs. . . .* The NHF recommends that patients maintain the use of concentrates or cryoprecipitates as prescribed by their physicians" (cited in IOM 1995:74). The French association was silent in public and in its communications to patients, leaving treatment decisions to physicians until, beginning in 1987, silence was no longer possible (Carricaburu 2000, Fillion 2009).[4] Hemophilia was expensive to treat, and those rare experts who urged them to switch to safer (and also cheaper) products were accused by French hemophiliacs of aiding and abetting government penny-pinching (Assemblée Nationale 1993:158).

In the late 1980s and early 1990s, hemophiliacs in both France and the United States slowly became engaged in the deadly game of crafting a response to AIDS. It was at this point that French and American strategies began to diverge. As Tarrow observes, "challengers are encouraged to take collective action when they have allies who can act as friends in court" (Tarrow 1998:79). French hemophiliacs were highly successful in cultivating influential allies among journalists, politically active gay men and, ultimately, in the courts; American hemophiliacs were not.

Mobilization

"Mobilizing structures"—social networks, institutions, and the connecting structures within and between them—are central to the birth and sustenance of social movements (Tarrow 1998:27). Hemophiliacs were brought together not only by formal interest-group associations but also by the exigencies of their disease, in hospitals where they could spend periods as long as a year, in treatment centers and, in France, in a network of boarding schools. Nevertheless, asserts Fillion, in France "the preexistence of a collectivity

---

[4] The reasons for associations' reluctance to speak out have been intensely scrutinized in the large literature on the blood crisis in France, in the U.S. IOM report, and in the few books on the blood affair the United States. We return to this question below in the context of interpreting patterns of mobilization.

dedicated to the defense of hemophiliacs (i.e., the AFH) was *unfavorable* to the mobilization of victims bent on accusation" (2009:139, emphasis added). Fillion describes in detail the intense "familial" relationships established almost from birth between the affected child, his parents, and their physician. "In this 'domestic' (at least one French observer described it as 'infantilizing') universe, everything conspired to create a traditional clinical model specific to hemophilia where the physician appeared as a figure at the same time authoritative and completely devoted, all powerful in her domain" (Fillion 2009:49).[5] These intense relationships extended beyond the immediate, quasi-domestic, circle to encompass the local blood bank (treatment centers in France were co-terminus with transfusion centers), blood donor associations, and their patrons. "Meetings of the AFH were often the occasion for physicians, parents and hemophilia patients, blood donors—sometimes even elected officials and local politicians—to celebrate the republican values of the French transfusion system" (Fillion 2009:135). These circumstances explain at least in part the extreme reluctance of the AFH to bring suit against Centre de Transfusion Sanguine (CTS) physicians ("Visit your doctor the day after a trial? Impossible!"), and, at the same time, many hemophiliacs' profound sense of betrayal when they learned of blood contamination: "I had the feeling, with Garretta, that the father had stabbed his son in the back" (cited by Fillion 2009:132).

Curative medicine (the *clinique* in French parlance) symbolized by the personal relationship between doctor and patient is culturally privileged in France; historically, the authority of doctors, combining "recognized knowledge, exclusive authority to pronounce on danger and risk, and privileged access to the state" was largely unquestioned (Nathanson 2007:222).[6] Medical experts in the United States enjoyed no comparable authority (see, e.g., Jasanoff 1990, Nathanson 2007). Each of the two national associations of hemophiliacs was shaped by the historical and cultural context in which it was formed and had its being. The French AFH was founded in 1955 by the foremost hematologist in France, also at that time head of the CNTS (a position he kept for the next thirty years), together with a wealthy hemophiliac. Although publicly positioned as an association of patients and their families, AFH was in fact driven from its beginning by physicians "who intervened

---

[5] The majority of French hemophilia doctors were women, and the patients, of course, were boys and men, introducing, Fillion suggests, complications of gender and sexuality into an already intense set of relationships.

[6] The status of public health was correspondingly weak (Steffen 1999:101, Chauveau 2011:185).

directly in its internal administration, managed its communications with the outside world, and were its interlocutors with the state" (Fillion 2009:124). Its American counterpart, in marked contrast, was founded (in 1948) by the parents of sons with hemophilia: "From the beginning, parents had power, largely because physicians had little to offer in the way of treatment or technical expertise; clinicians were virtually powerless" (Resnik 1999:34). Over time, the NHF—much like other chronic disease associations in the United States (Best 2019)—evolved into a remarkably effective grassroots lobbying organization, advocating successfully for state and federal funding for hemophilia research and treatment. With advances in technology (e.g., the advent of an easily administered blood-clotting factor), physicians gained greater power within the NHF but never to the exclusion of lay leadership. Even so, this power came under serious attack when technology bit back in the form of AIDS.

France

Hemophiliacs' engagement with AIDS in France began in 1987: quietly and discretely on the part of AFH, publicly and (at least as perceived by its targets) aggressively by a small but militant group dissatisfied with AFH's "insider" approach. The first steps taken by the AFH was to write a series of letters to the then minister of health, Michèle Barzach, calling attention to the plight of French hemophiliacs (the focus was on families whose principal breadwinner had died of AIDS) and asking for assistance, comparable to what would be offered to victims of flood or terrorism. "There was no thought of accusation. The request was for a gesture of solidarity on behalf of victims of technical progress and not for compensation for faults of which the association was not yet fully conscious" (Fillion 2009:145). The AFH approached members of Parliament with the same end in view—again personally, quietly, and discretely. The impact of HIV on persons with hemophilia was framed in these early efforts as an accident—"the blind effect of nature" (Goffman, cited in Stone 1989:284). Over time—receiving no response they deemed satisfactory and under pressure from the association's members—the tone of these letters became more severe, directly invoking the responsibility of the state. (Barzach had suggested AFH bring suit against their doctors and the blood centers, a strategy AFH deemed directly contrary to its members interests, "who would have to live with [these persons] all their lives" [Hermitte 1996:349]). In March 1989, his patience exhausted, the president of AFH (himself infected with HIV) gave an interview to *Le Monde*, published under the title "AIDS: Hemophiliacs Give an Ultimatum to the Government." Our association, said the president, Bruno de Langre, "is not seeking a polemic or an 'affair,' " but, "if we are not heard, we will attack the State" (March 25, 1989).

Within the state—or at least within its health ministerial cabinet—de Langre was heard almost immediately. In a memo to his minister dated five days after the *Le Monde* piece and labeled "explosive," the responsible cabinet member wrote: "The solidarity of those in charge [i.e., political and administrative health authorities in collaboration with the AFH] accomplished through silence is splintering now that the facts are being progressively brought to the attention of the public and, principally, the victims" (FNA, March 30, 1989). In other words, the AFH—heretofore the state's "reasonable" partner in contrast to much more demanding victims represented by militant "outsiders"—was threatening to go public. Pushed by this threat—lent credibility by increasing press attention to the plight of hemophiliacs—the government announced a *fonds de solidarité* (literally, a solidarity fund) funded in part by the government and in part by insurers and, specifically, with no implication of state responsibility.[7] By the time this gesture was made (August 1989) it satisfied no one (Hermitte 1996:322). Apart from the modest amounts proposed, the exclusion of the transfused and the seropositive (only hemophiliacs were eligible and only those with AIDS), and the obligation that acceptance entailed not to go to the courts, the element that most angered the militants among French hemophiliacs was the state's refusal to acknowledge its responsibility for their tragedy.[8]

Jean Péron-Garvanoff founded the ADP (Association de Défense des Polytransfusés, or Association for Defense of the Multiply Transfused) in 1987, when hemophiliacs first became aware of their "collective catastrophe"

[7] Riedmattan (1992) attributes the creation of the *fonds* at least in part to insurers' refusal to insure blood banks against what they anticipated would be the enormous costs—amounting to billions of francs—if each person who acquired HIV through transfusion (many more than hemophiliacs) were to sue individually. On July 1, 1989, a French court had awarded 2.3 million francs, payable by the blood bank, to a woman who acquired HIV subsequent to transfusion as a result of an automobile accident (58). Evin cabinet documents show that Garretta was insistent that insurers would not cover the blood banks and had been lobbying for state-funded indemnity since mid-1988 or earlier.

[8] The refusal of direct responsibility on the part of both the health administration (the DGS) and the government's political arm (the cabinet) is a constant theme in health cabinet documents from 1988 through 1990. See Chapter 4.

(Hermitte 1996:349).[9] Garvanoff—a jazz pianist from a large family of Bulgarian gypsy origin living on the outskirts of Paris—was a hemophiliac as were his two brothers (both of whom, as well as Garvanoff himself, later died of AIDS). The apocryphal story is that Garvanoff learned of the threat to hemophiliacs in the mid-1980s at a cocktail party thrown by his doctor, Jean-Pierre Allain, who had invited him and a colleague to entertain the guests (Riedmatten 1992). But Garvanoff had a prepared mind. Alerted in 1983 by the French media to potential contamination of the blood supply in the United States, Garvanoff sought confirmation from American friends; the overheard conversation at the cocktail party both confirmed what he already knew and made clear that the problem was not confined to the United States. For the next six years, Garvanoff—first on his own and later with the help of HIV-affected family and friends organized as the ADP—besieged the AFH, politicians of all persuasions and at all levels from the French president on down, parliamentarians, blood bankers and, ultimately, of most importance, the press with detailed information and demands for redress. Garvanoff's letter to the new health minister shortly after the latter took office in 1988 accusing his predecessors of having "buried the scandal" was cited earlier. Prior to eruption of the blood affair into the public arena in 1991, responses to letters from the ADP ranged from rude to polite to promises of follow-up that failed to materialize (Riedmattan 1992, Hermitte 1996, Fillion 2009). Evin cabinet documents make clear that AFH was regarded as the government's privileged interlocutor; the competition from their radical flank both contributed to AFH's aura of "reasonableness" and was effective in ratcheting up pressure on officials extremely reluctant to assume any responsibility for the problems of persons with hemophilia (Fillion 2009:151).[10] On the grounds of this failure to publicly accept responsibility, Garvanoff and the ADP rejected compensation from the *fonds* and sought restitution from the courts. "Causal politics," as Stone observes, "is centrally concerned with moving interpretations of a situation from the realm of accident" to the realm of human control (1989:284). Garvanoff and his colleagues were

[9] Once a test became available in 1985, French physicians urged their hemophiliac patients to be tested (and then reassured them when the test was positive) (Fillion 2009). There is some evidence of less pressure toward testing of hemophiliacs by their U.S. providers due to fear of discrimination (Resnik oral history archives).

[10] "Radical flank" is a term of art in sociology that refers to "interactive processes involving radical and moderate factions of social movements . . . . They result in detrimental and/or beneficial impacts of radical group actions upon the reputations and effectiveness of more moderate collective actors" (Haines 1984).

highly successful in moving the interpretation of HIV in the blood supply from tragic accident to deliberate intent, a toxic mix of economic greed and ministerial cover-up.

ADP was not a support group for hemophiliacs, nor did it engage in street-level protests. Its tactics were, as Fillion points out, unprecedented in France: first, to take its demands to court and, second, to "instrumentalize" the media, not only breaking with the insider strategy adopted by AFH but also engaging in what were in context highly innovative forms of collective mobilization.[11] When lobbying the AFH directly and letter-writing proved ineffective in generating action on behalf of hemophiliacs infected with HIV, Garvanoff and his colleagues turned to the courts, targeting first the CNTS for—as it finally came down to—"merchandising fraud" (*tromperie sur les qualités substantielles des produits sanguins*).[12] Very quickly additional targets were added (most notably the National Health Laboratory [Laboratoire National de la Santé], unambiguously, as compared to CNTS, an arm of the state) and additional legal theories were invoked (e.g., non-assistance to persons in danger, poisoning, and—at the extreme—crimes against humanity) (Hermitte 1996:350). The charge retained by the prosecutors who brought the combined complaints of multiple hemophiliacs to trial in the summer of 1992 was that of "merchandising fraud."[13]

French public prosecutors did not take cognizance of the blood affair on their own. To all appearances (as filtered through the media) after the 1985 brouhaha over testing, the blood system was back to normal, and there appeared no reason for the courts to intervene (Hermitte 1996:347). The blood affair was launched only when—in the spring of 1988 after multiple setbacks—militant hemophiliacs convinced the public prosecutorial system to take their case. To understand how this system (the *parquet*) got

[11] Advocates employed a combination of what Kitschelt would have called *assimilative* (insider) and *confrontational* (outsider) tactics drawn from an international repertoire of collective action (including the actions of gay militants in the United States) (Kitschelt 1986). As Tilly observed, "changing interest, opportunity, and organization influence [ordinary people's] prevailing modes of collective action" (Tilly 1986:8).

[12] For a detailed account of Garvanoff's difficulties in finding lawyers to take his case, see Kramer 1993. We will return to the question of how Garvanoff and ADP ruptured traditional French perspectives on law and society, but a brief quote from Cohen-Tanugi will give an idea: "Traditionally the French have not really believed in the relevance of the law for resolving the major political, economic or social conflicts which grip the nation, and French society manifests a fair amount of tolerance for failure to respect the rule of law" (Cohen-Tanugi 1996:269).

[13] The French case was grounded in a 1905 law against merchandising fraud, extended in 1978 to explicitly cover all medical products and services (Kramer 1993). See Chapter 6 for a detailed description of the differences between France and the United States in legal frameworks and arguments pertaining to blood cases.

into the act, we must introduce the concept of *"partie civile."* French legal procedure allows individuals (e.g., individual hemophiliacs) and recognized associations (e.g., ADP) to demand recovery as, essentially, third parties (victims) harmed by the actions of a defendant (in the present case, actors in the blood system). Among the more consequential outcomes of being accepted by the *parquet* as a *partie civile* is that collection of the relevant evidence immediately becomes the responsibility of the state. By the time the blood affair broke into the public arena in the spring of 1991, the investigator appointed by the presiding judge—a lieutenant-colonel in charge of criminal investigations at the Gendarmerie Nationale—had been at his work for three years (Kramer 1993).

Among the many recipients of Garvanoff's letters were the editors of France's major newspapers, popular and "serious," left and right.[14] In their engagement with the media, Garvanoff and the ADP adopted what Fillion describes as "transformative" modes of public action: "mobilization of the media in order to arouse public indignation in favor of the victims" of contaminated blood (2009:149). Acting in effect as a "door-to-door salesman," Garvanoff solicited the press irrespective of format or political persuasion to convince journalists not only of "scandal" but also of moral responsibility on the part of government that mere compensation without the acknowledgment of fault would not satisfy. Before 1991, with the exception of presidents of the AFH, Garvanoff was the public face of the hemophiliac tragedy in France. Much like Asterix the Gaul, beloved by the French as a potent symbol of man against the machine, Garvanoff "incarnated the straight-talking man without connections who fought the establishment for years almost alone to unlock the scandal" (Marchetti 2010:155).

Paris is the center of the French political universe, of its elite medical and intellectual universe and, consequently, of its journalistic universe. Journalists go where the stories are, and the big stories—medical, political, and those that blur the lines between—emanate (or at least are perceived to emanate) from Paris. All of France's major newspapers are headquartered in Paris as are its television stations. Until the early 1980s medical journalism insofar as it appeared in the mainstream press (as opposed to professional organs) acted essentially as a handmaiden to the medical profession, transmitting physicians' pronouncements with little change or comment; further, transmission was heavily dominated by the major afternoon daily

---

[14] France's major newspapers have distinct and popularly well-understood political flavors.

paper *Le Monde*.[15] Transformation of this journalistic landscape began in the early 1980s, resulting in an increased politicization of medical journalism, intense competition within the field, and if not the loss altogether, then a substantial softening of *Le Monde*'s commanding position.[16]

Marchetti argues that the success of Garvanoff and the ADP in gaining attention from the press was contingent on the increasing internal competitiveness of French medical journalism: "Hemophiliacs and their lawyers would probably have had less success in mobilizing the media if medical journalists in the major media outlets (*médias grands publics*) were not so strongly opposed to one another" (2010:100). *Le Monde* in particular had powerful incentives for the competitive amplification of political crisis. By the time Casteret published her incendiary article in *L'Événement du jeudi*, *Le Monde* had been covering this story for several years: "The Scandal of Hemophiliacs" under the byline of Jean Yves Nau, its principal medical journalist, was published two years earlier in April 1989.[17] The paper's reaction to Casteret's putative "scoop" was, first, to downplay her revelations and, second, to enlarge the scope of responsibility from actors it characterized as lower level "scapegoats" like Garretta to health ministers and prime ministers. From early in the AIDS epidemic the journalists of not only *Le Monde* but also those of the other major papers and TV channels had cultivated close relationships with scientists, cabinet members, and health officials; using these sources, they "created" stories, outing key documents often before their publication or official release: "Very often . . . they knew certain '*dossiers*' better than the principals" (Marchetti 2010:101).[18]

Fillion contextualizes hemophiliacs' campaign more broadly within "a profound evolution of relationships within the public sphere at the same time

---

[15] French media conservatism prior to 1980 is confirmed in these comments by Stanley Hoffman, then professor of the Civilization of France at Harvard: "And the media are remarkably respectful; television is the instrument of the state, and the press shows little enthusiasm for investigative reporting—the pro-majority press respects sacred cows, the opposition press prefers principled denunciation to empirical scrutiny." (Hoffmann 1980:viii).

[16] The reasons for this transformation are complex: politicization of medicine itself centered around the cost of medical care, the shift from state-run to commercial television channels, and changes in journalistic staff at *Le Monde* and other major papers bringing in younger, more aggressive, more "political" left-wing journalists with medical training (Champagne and Marchetti 1994, Marchetti 2010).

[17] It is important to note that Casteret had called attention to the HIV/blood problem in an article published in 1983 in a popular medical journal and had published "La tragédie des hémophiles" ("The Tragedy of Hemophiliacs") in a daily paper, *L'Express*, in 1987. Not until she was able to transform "tragedy" into "scandal" did Casteret catch on.

[18] Saul's analysis of French journalistic coverage of the blood affair also emphasizes its intense competitiveness (2004:96).

as collective mobilization" around identity-based claims (2009:150). In the United States, identity-based collective mobilization against AIDS centered on gay men, leaving little space for hemophiliacs in the public sphere and, indeed, creating profound disincentives for mobilization by hemophiliacs. As we noted in an earlier chapter, although gay associations expanded in France during the early 1980s, they were largely absent from the AIDS political sphere. When gay men did begin to mobilize politically—Act Up-Paris was founded in 1989—their first public protests were in support of hemophiliacs, close to the inverse of what happened in the United States. In competition with its well-established, but deliberately not gay-identified rival, AIDES, Act Up-Paris used the blood affair to make its mark on the political stage—to "build its public and political capital" (Pinell 2002:248). Act Up-Paris was small, militant, and antiestablishment; its tactics modeled on its American counterpart. Framing the blood affair as the responsibility of a "murderous" government and engaging in highly in-your-face actions (e.g., splattering blood, using their bodies to block the street) was totally in keeping with its goal to become as visually important as possible. From Act Up-Paris' perspective, the already notorious blood affair was a gift and an opportunity. In exploiting this opportunity to the hilt they—along with the journalists who rewarded Act Up's media-savvy tactics with front-page coverage—were key elements in popular adoption and amplification of intentional wrongdoing as the dominant causal story in France. We emphasize that intense competition *within* their respective fields for space and attention in the public arena was common to *both* the Paris journalists *and* the AIDS militants. This internal—within field—competition was critical not only to these actors' initial mobilization but also to the accompanying cycle of amplification, sustained at high pitch for almost two years (see Figure 1.1).

United States

The militant wing of French hemophiliacs played an outside game, making a clear break with their voluntary association in almost every dimension of tactics and strategy. American militants were split. In the words of a participant with feet in both militant and more establishment camps, "What we planned was an inside revolution [i.e., upending the agenda of the NHF]. And in the meantime, someone else started an outside revolution" with the aim [from this actor's perspective] of destroying the NHF altogether" (oral history, Resnik Archives, May 1, 1997).[19] "Outside" in this case meant out-side the NHF, not "outside" in the public sphere. Even the most militant of U.S. hemophiliacs engaged primarily in "insider" strategies, actions in the courts and lobbying government officials and members of Congress not public demonstrations in the style of Act Up. Neither the establishment nor the militant camps, in what was, to a large extent, an internal struggle, captured the interest of the American national media to an extent remotely comparable with the sustained, even obsessive, media attention accorded to their French counterparts.

In the late 1980s, when Garvanoff was pounding on the doors of journalists, officials, and members of Parliament, and the French press as well as the courts had begun to recognize there was a problem with hemophiliacs, the United States was confronting a healthcare crisis generated by the increasing numbers and increasing medical costs of persons with AIDS. Gay rights or-ganization and their allies, state and local officials, members of Congress, the National Association of Public Hospitals, the National AIDS Commission, and, of critical importance, the press converged on the proposition that AIDS had produced "a crisis in the delivery of essential health services" and that some form of "disaster" relief was necessary. The National Commission on AIDS created in the summer of 1989 "urged Congress to take action and provide disaster relief for AIDS services" (Chambré 2006:104).[20] The re-sult was the Kennedy-Hatch bill (later renamed the Ryan White Care Act) passed in 1990 with overwhelming support both in the House and Senate. Congressional provision of "money to help people who were bound together not by age or income or disability but by a virus" (Chambré 2006:92) was an unprecedented act, made possible by the persistent efforts of gay rights or-ganizations and their allies in cities and states hard hit by the AIDS epidemic (Bayer and Kirp 1992).

Public attention is a scare resource (Hilgartner and Bosk 1988) as is the work of mobilization and organization required for collective action. Confronted by what was widely portrayed as imminent collapse of the

---

[19] Unless otherwise indicated, interviews from the Resnik Archives are with hemophiliacs either presently (at the time of interview) or formerly active in advocacy organizations on their behalf.

[20] It may be banal to point out that France has a national health service that covers the costs of hospital and ambulatory care. Nevertheless, this was a critical difference in the context within which the AIDS epidemic in the two countries unfolded. A crisis in the provision of health services was not a salient element of the political context in France. Indeed, their dependence on these extremely ex-pensive services was one of the initial barriers to mobilization of persons with hemophilia in France against the government, and some even suggested that government warnings about blood products were because the government was a cheapskate and didn't want to pay for these products.

healthcare system, there was little public space in the United States of the late 1980s for persons with hemophilia. The Ryan White Act was named for a young boy with hemophilia who was excluded from school because he had AIDS, causing public outrage; but Ryan White was a poster boy for deserving "innocent children," not for hemophiliacs, enabling advocates to link AIDS with "a population whose image was highly sympathetic and in stark contrast to the image of gay men and injection drug users" (Donovan 2001:61). Not only was there little room in the public sphere for persons with hemophilia and their families, but also hemophiliacs themselves were extremely reluctant to enter that sphere; they had no more desire to be associated with gay men and injection drug users than did members of Congress. Asked about connections with gay groups, a former president of the NHF responded: "Very little of that occurred. . . . [First] nobody with hemophilia wanted anyone to think they might have gotten the disease because they had a gay relationship. [Second] I guess people with hemophilia recognized the prejudice that was given to people who were gay with AIDS and didn't want any part of that either" (oral history, Resnik Archives, May 1, 1997). Highly publicized attacks on Ryan White in 1985 and on the Ray family in 1987 brought that prejudice home: "Many men who had been open about having hemophilia began to retreat . . . into a private world of their blood brothers and their families" (Resnik 1999:137).[21]

The tactic of invisibility (the former NHF president cited above referred to it as "hiding our heads in the sand") was starkly illustrated by the NHF's constituency's response to a modest effort on its part in the late 1980s to develop a "White Paper" "discussing the fact that hemophiliacs got AIDS" (Resnik 1999:155):

Our board and our chapters resoundingly voted it down. I shouldn't say resoundingly. The board was divided on it, but the chapters, when they saw this white paper, just got up in arms and said, you can't do this, we have people living in this community, if they're exposed their house could be destroyed, this will happen, that will happen, they'll be kicked out of school. . . . So, this white paper, then, never saw the light of day. It's

---

[21] The Ray family with three hemophiliac boys were not only hounded out of school but also their house in Florida was torched by arsonists, forcing them to move. Discrimination and fear of being identified as gay were issues for French persons with hemophilia as well, leading to concealment both of their disease and of HIV-positive status. Discrimination was denounced by the French government in 1988, and there is little evidence of a strong impact on mobilization in France.

important to point that out, because that was really the mentality of this whole community. (oral history, Resnik Archives, May 1, 1997)[22]

Highly publicized stigma and discrimination, reluctance to be identified with gays, and a public sphere heavily focused on the larger AIDS epidemic led to marked delay both in their recognition of collective interests and in mobilization of hemophiliacs in the United States as compared with France.[23] Change came about in part due to the increased visibility of sickness and death among friends and family members but also—perhaps surprisingly— due to the role of the CDC in bringing men with hemophilia together in what rapidly developed into a strong—if somewhat limited—protest movement. Following a lobbying campaign by the NHF, the U.S. Congress in 1986 "appropriated supplemental funding for 'risk reduction' in the hemophilia community to the Centers for Disease Control (CDC), with the understanding that funds would be distributed to the treatment centers through Maternal and Child Health's Hemophilia Program" (Resnik 1999:143). The CDC's agenda—focused on confronting AIDS directly through testing and education for "safe sex"—was quite different than that of the NHF, and the CDC now controlled the funds.[24] Nevertheless, the CDC may not have anticipated exactly how those funds would be used: "[The] revolution that occurred within the hemophilia community in the 1990s was really as a result of work that the NHF was able to get the CDC to fund. The NHF brought together a series of focus groups on the state of the hemophilia community— the impact of AIDS on people with hemophilia in the early 1990s" (oral history, Resnik Archives, May 1, 1997).

The transformation of CDC-funded focus groups into an organized protest movement of angry young men happened very rapidly, galvanized by the opportunity these groups presented to share—often for the first

[22] Stigma went well beyond the most publicized cases. Elaine DePrince describes how in the late 1980s her two small sons with hemophilia and AIDS were "cruelly harassed" and "excluded from neighborhood play," their car damaged, and the like (1997:175).

[23] Hemophiliacs in France were tested as soon as blood tests for AIDS became available in France in 1985 (Carricaburu 2000). Oral history interviews suggest that in the United States treatment clinics for hemophiliacs may have been reluctant to test due to fear that their clients would become uninsurable.

[24] As late as 1990, the immediate past president of the NHF reflected on the organization's internal conflict: "There's this major battle between whether we should be—we as the Foundation—should be letting the public know that hemophilia and AIDS really are connected. . . . I don't think people really have made the link, that a lot of people with hemophilia are HIV positive. That's good if you want to hide from discrimination. It's very bad if you want to try and deal with really what the hemophilia community is dealing with today" (oral history, 1990, Resnik archives).

time—detailed information on the origins of their infection: the connection between blood, hemophilia, and AIDS.[25] In 1990, the U.S. Congress—specifically the House Subcommittee on Oversight and Investigations under the leadership of John Dingell (D-MI)—held hearings on "Blood Supply Safety" (U.S. House of Representatives 1990).[26] Dingell's opening statement set the tone: "This inquiry has its roots in the early 1980s when the blood industry and the Government failed to prevent transfusion of thousands of pints of blood and blood products infected with the AIDS virus" (p. 1). In the course of testimony from the executive director of the NHF, the FDA, and blood experts, as well as in documents submitted to the Subcommittee, the facts of blood contamination in the early 1980s and of failed efforts to protect the blood supply and blood products were laid bare. Press coverage of these hearings was minimal, relegated to inside pages and treated by and large as old news. Nevertheless, a few hemophiliacs paid attention: "This is all documented . . . you can obtain this information—it's all public—from the Committee of Oversight and Investigation that took place regarding AIDS and the blood safety, blood safety in the country" (oral history, Resnik Archives, September 19, 1991). And another participant reflected: "Boy these were guys that were pissed off. They had the ability to get together and start to dig through documents early on" (oral history, Resnick Archives, July 15, 1997).

The rapid conversion of anger into organized protest was eloquently described by a close observer and sometime participant who later became the president of NHF:

> The anger was addressed largely toward the manufacturers for giving them this contaminated product, but was also . . . directed toward the NHF, for not providing all the facts in a balanced way as they saw it in the early 1980s, and it was directed against their docs, against their treatment centers. So, all of this came out because we had the ability to get people together in a room at the same time, get phone numbers out, telephone trees got set up, networks were established, there were a couple of other meetings. MANN

[25] This statement is documented in oral histories of several participants (Resnik oral history archives).

[26] An article in the Minneapolis *Star Tribune* on December 9, 1990, states this hearing was triggered by Gilbert Gaul's Pulitzer Prize–winning articles in the *Philadelphia Inquirer* exposing the "'billion-dollar business' of blood and how it is bought and sold in a virtually unregulated market" (Joseph Feldschuh and Doron Weber, *Star Tribune*, December 9, 1990, 25A.). Gaul's five-part series appeared originally in September 1989 (see Chapter 2).

[Men's Advocacy Network of the NHF] developed, and it was clear that it was moving very very rapidly throughout 1991. By early '92 the organization was approaching somewhat of a crisis because MANN had become powerful very quickly, and all of the men who were powerful in MANN were men who had not previously been associated with the NHF. (oral history, Resnik Archives, May 1, 1997)

MANN rapidly split into a (relatively) moderate wing advocating change from within the organization—an "inside revolution"—and a radical flank wanting an "outside revolution" that would overturn NHF altogether. The moderate wing ultimately prevailed, overturning the traditional leadership of NHF and turning it into a strongly consumer-driven organization, but at the cost of intense internal turmoil created by the "outside" revolutionaries, the Committee of Ten Thousand (COTT) and the HIV Peer Association (PEER) in the years 1991–1993.

Nevertheless, in a classic radical-flank effect pointed out by a person closely involved, "one function that these groups [COTT and PEER] have served is that being outside the system, it's actually been effective having a group that has less boundaries in terms of like the NHF who is a more of an established system . . . . To have these groups outside where they had a lot more leeway, like in terms of doing protests. Bringing issues up, railing, you know, *actually it was quite effective in getting a number of issues pushed forward*" (oral history, Resnik Archives, May 1, 1997, emphasis added). Among the critical actions pushed by COTT and PEER were (1) a class action lawsuit against the blood products industry; (2) a congressional investigation into contamination of the blood supply; and (3) federally funded compensation for HIV-infected hemophiliacs and their families.

In sharp contrast to what happened in France where the crisis that stemmed from hemophiliacs' recognition of their contamination by tainted blood products moved rapidly into the public sphere, the same crisis in the United States remained almost entirely internal to the small community of hemophiliacs and their families. In closed testimony before the IOM Committee to Study HIV Transmission Through Blood Products (1994) and in congressional hearings on the question of compensation (1996, see Chapter 7), persons with hemophilia and their survivors framed their grievances in ways that resembled the French—their suffering was not an accident but "premediated murder" motivated by corporate greed—but also departed from them in ways that appear intended to portray hemophiliacs as uniquely deserving: "[My wife] was a true innocent victim of the AIDS epidemic, as are all hemophiliacs" (U.S. House of Representatives 1996:140). In these testimonies the sufferers are uniformly presented as embedded in "families" with children sometimes adding their voices to those of the parent; witnesses present themselves as God-fearing "citizens" with an emphasis on church attendance; they present themselves as taxpayers, "refusing to let [their families] be a burden to the Government" (U.S. House of Representatives 1996:145). It is difficult not to interpret these statements as intended to insulate persons with hemophilia from the dual stigmas of "welfare" dependent and gay.

However hemophilacs' grievances were framed, they gained almost no traction in the public sphere. There was little or no press coverage either of the hemophilia community's internal struggles or of their claims of betrayal and injustice and no official public recognition of these claims until the late 1990s, following publication of the IOM report. This vacuum is attributable in part to the same contextual variables mentioned earlier: limited space on the public stage and its dominance by the larger AIDS epidemic among gay men and injection drug users.[27] Insofar as there was public concern as reflected in newspaper reports it was with the current (in 1990) safety of the blood supply not with the plight of hemophiliacs. The all but exclusive dominance of technological perspectives in the U.S. response is captured in Keshavjee, Weiser, and Kleinman's comment on the IOM report: "Instead of addressing the moral questions raised by the contamination of the blood supply, the Report converted the suffering of the hemophilia community into policy analysis and an exercise in the study of better management and regulatory oversight" (2001:1089).

Reflections

There are striking parallels between France and the United States in how hemophiliacs engaged with their condition before the advent of AIDS and even—within limits—in how they responded to the tragedy of blood contamination. The world of hemophiliacs in both countries was characterized by intense and continuing relationships with providers of care and—since the

---

[27] As we will describe more fully in the next chapter, a third variable may have been the success of blood industry defendants in preventing most lawsuits by hemophiliacs and blood transfusion recipients from going to trial, with the attendant publicity that such trials might have attracted.

advent of easily accessible blood-clotting technology in the 1970s—by dependence on a multinational blood industry. And protest in both countries was shaped in part by the emergence of a radical flank at odds with their traditional organizations, claiming betrayal and demanding compensation. There, however, the parallels cease. Mobilization was substantially earlier in France due in part to absence of the overt stigma and discrimination against hemophiliacs with AIDS that made Americans extremely reluctant to come forward.[28] Second, although their tactics were different, both the Association Française des Hémophiles (AFH) and the Association de Défense des Polytransfusés (ADP) moved rapidly to demand action by the state, and the ADP's suit as *partie civile*—giving the "radicals" access to the full investigative powers of the judicial system—was accepted by the court in 1988. COTT did not approach national legislators until 1993 (in the first year of the Clinton administration), and its plea for a congressional investigation was turned down. In 1995, hemophiliacs' class action suit (also led by members of COTT) against the pharmaceutical industry was rejected by the U.S. Court of Appeals for the Seventh Circuit (*In the Matter of Rhone-Poulenc Rorer* 1995).[29]

But the most consequential differences between France and the United States were, first, the reciprocal engagement of hemophiliacs and the media in France and, second, the sustained moral outrage (reflected first in the media and quickly thereafter in statements and actions of French government officials) that followed Casteret's revelations in April 1991. Given their fears of stigma and discrimination, hemophiliacs in the United States actively shied away from the public attention that engagement with the media would bring; hemophiliacs have been marginalized in intellectual discourse on AIDS in this country; and there was (and is) no evidence of the moral outrage at their fate (amplified not only by the media but also by diverse forms of collective action) that resulted in political crisis and policy transformation in France.

Muffled and Absent Voices

Persons with hemophilia and their sexual partners were not, of course, the only victims of toxic blood, and HIV is hardly the only virus that blood

---

[28] In the first years of AIDS in France, hemophiliacs had also been reluctant to come forward in part for the same reasons articulated in the United States and because they were acutely conscious of hemophilia treatment's cost to the country's national health insurance program. In the late 1980s, parties of both left and right in France united against Le Pen's proposals for institutionalized discrimination against persons with AIDS making nondiscrimination the clear policy of the state. This policy was forcefully articulated by ministers and in the press (see, e.g., Got 1989).

[29] As described in Chapter 6, a settlement with the pharmaceutical industry was reached in 1997.

may transmit. But hemophiliacs were privileged not only by their status as "innocent victims" (unlike injection drug users, who were also infected by contaminated blood) but also by their "mobilizing structures," that is, associations, treatment centers, specialized schools, and recreational venues, that brought them together prior to the advent of AIDS. Although individuals who acquired HIV through whole blood transfusion were two-to-three times more numerous than hemophiliacs, they had far more difficulty in gaining recognition. In both France and the United States transfusion recipients were "isolated across the country without anything in common except their suffering and their misery" (*Le Monde*, January 29, 1990). Nevertheless, due in large part to the active engagement of a member of the French Senate, an association on behalf of persons with transfusion-acquired AIDS was formed in early 1990 and lobbied successfully for the inclusion of this category of victims in the French compensation legislation passed in December 1991. Their American counterparts were less fortunate. Despite the best efforts of an American Senator, James Jeffords (R-VT), opposition to the inclusion of transfusion victims in comparable U.S. legislation not only by its Senate sponsors but also by the NHF on the grounds the inclusion of transfusees would sink the bill in Congress meant persons with transfusion-acquired HIV infection were left out. "Congress still isn't hearing much from constituents about the issue. These folks just aren't well organized, and it's very difficult to get support for a bill without that kind of grass-roots activity," explained a congressional staffer (*Washington Post*, January 2, 2001).

More surprising perhaps, since not only were they well organized but also had excellent political connections throughout the country, was the silence of France's blood donor associations: they "said nothing, or almost nothing, about the affair of contaminated blood" (Chauveau 2007:711). In her comprehensive study of the blood affair in France, Chauveau advances several hypotheses to account for this silence. First, from the perspective of these associations, donation of French blood and contamination were contradictions in terms. French blood was pure by definition. An attack on French blood and, by extension, on the French blood system was almost sacrilegious;[30] it amounted to an attack on French society itself. Second, much like associations of hemophiliacs in both France and the United States, French blood donor associations were closely allied not only ideologically but also materially with the French transfusion centers (CTS) that both collected and

[30] The word "sacrilege" was used by Senator Henri Caillavet in an interview with the newspaper *Le Figaro* in late 1991 to explain what the reporter described as a "delay" in recognition of the blood crisis. Caillavet founded the French association In Defense of Transfusees.

processed blood. "It was difficult for donors, as for hemophiliacs, to be critical of those who allowed their associations to survive" (Chauveau 2011:178). Finally, blood donor associations were far more concerned with what they regarded as the totally unacceptable transition in the status of blood from sacred substance to regulated pharmaceutical drug required by France's membership in the European Union, a transition already delayed that was finally accomplished in 1993. Among the consequences of this transition and of the reform of France's blood system that followed upon the blood crisis was a much reduced role in blood system activities for these associations (Chauveau 2011:177).

PART II

BLOOD EPISTEMOLOGY

Prologue

Epistemology is "the study or a theory of the nature and grounds of knowledge especially with reference to its limits and validity." Interrogation of "knowledge" about the blood affair—and especially the limits and validity of that knowledge—began simultaneously with recognition of the HIV-blood nexus in the public sphere. This interrogation had begun privately in the early 1980s among experts in the medicine and science of blood. Our purpose here, however, is to explore and compare the multiple public accounts—the Greek chorus of fact and interpretation by the media, the courts, committees, commissions, political bodies, and academia—that succeeded popular recognition. Both chronology and the interweaving of country and chorus members are somewhat arbitrary.

We begin with the highly public, highly mediatized Paris trial of blood banks and health officials, in part because litigation began early in France and was central to hemophiliacs' mobilization strategy and to the social production of the blood crisis. There were trials in the United States but nothing comparable to the *auto-da-fé* that played out in France in the summer of 1992. We turn next (in Chapter 7) to the question of compensation. Both countries offered financial compensation to HIV-infected hemophiliacs, France much earlier and more generously, the United States ten years later and more parsimoniously. Extensive political (in the form of parliamentary and congressional hearings) and media (far more in France than in the United States) commentary accompanied these actions. Finally (as described in Chapter 8), in France both the initial official and semi-official "reports" on the blood affair were published in 1991–1992 and were integral to the social production of crisis. The sole comparable report in the United States was not published until 1995. We have elected to discuss these reports together (along with the 1993 report from the French Assemblée Nationale) since they come nearest to parallel official accounts of the blood affair.

6

Litigation

France

"Culpable but not responsible."[1] Within a year and a half of Casteret's article in *L'Événement du jeudi*, there appeared in print no less than four more or less authoritative, more or less damning narratives of the French blood story: the official "Lucas" report in the fall of 1991; the report of the French Senate published in June 1992; Casteret's book-length elaboration of her original story; and *Le Monde* reporter Laurent Greilsamer's equally lengthy account of the "contaminated blood trial" before the *"tribunal de grande instance de Paris,"* extending over six weeks in the hot summer of 1992.[2] The principal story line varied very little across these accounts: motivated by economic greed, blood banks and government health officials made conscious decisions that resulted in the deaths from AIDS of (to that date) over a thousand hemophiliacs in France and infection with the HIV virus of many more.[3] Very quickly, this tale of greed and betrayal became the accepted narrative of the blood affair in France.

Among these stories, Greilsamer's was by far the most dramatic, as was—by all accounts—the trial itself. There were, at the trial's outset (June 24, 1992), "some 50 lawyers, an equal number of journalists, 20 gendarmes, the *'parties civiles'* (the hemophiliacs) and the public, [and] the 'black robes' (judges)," not to speak of the four individuals accused, crammed into a courtroom never intended to accommodate a crowd of that size.[4] Through the open windows, members of Act Up-Paris outside the courthouse could be heard

---

[1] Assertion by former French health minister, 1991.
[2] *"Tribunal de grande instance"* (TGI) is the French court of first resort.
[3] Whatever the reality may have been, in these accusatory accounts little distinction was made between the motives of blood banks and ministers.
[4] Many accounts of this trial have been published. We rely on Greilsamer's detailed narrative, which includes the prosecutor's opening statement (*réquisitoire*), a frequently verbatim day-by-day account of the trial itself, and the court's final judgment. Both the opening statement and the final judgment are recorded verbatim.

The Social Production of Crisis. Constance A. Nathanson and Henri Bergeron, Oxford University Press.
© Oxford University Press 2023. DOI: 10.1093/oso/9780197682487.003.0006

shouting "Murderer," "Assassin," a refrain they would keep up over the entire length of the trial.[5] The leading actors in this drama—the accused—were Michel Garretta, former director of the Centre Nationale de Transfusion Sanguine (CNTS); Jean-Pierre Allain, its former medical director; Jacques Roux, former director of the Direction Générale de la Santé (DGS), an administrative arm of the French Ministry of Health responsible for public health; and Robert Netter, former head of the Laboratoire Nationale de la Santé (LNS), the nearest equivalent at the time to a French FDA. All four defendants were trained as physicians. As we will describe more fully below, Garretta and Allain were accused of fraud and Roux and Netter of "non-assistance to persons in danger."

The trial had its origins in 1988, when small groups of hemophiliacs, acting as "*parties civiles*," were—after at least a year of fruitless attempts—finally successful in having their complaints accepted by the prosecutorial system in Paris.[6] This happened, observed their lawyer, Georges Holleaux, "at a time when there was total disbelief [that the blood system could be at fault for infecting hemophiliacs with HIV] and only a few relevant articles had appeared in the press" (Greilsamer 1992:94). Over the next four years, additional plaintiffs came forward as *parties civiles* (numbering at least sixty by the time of the trial) under the aegis of Garvanoff's ADP (the Association de Défense des Polytransfusées). In March 1992, the instructing judge, Mme. Sabine Foulon, joined the complaints together as grounded in a single set of facts: the contamination of the individual plaintiff and/or family members with HIV by blood products the plaintiff had received.

The complexities and eventual legal ramifications of this litigation were profound and understandable only in the context of first, a legal climate long favorable to persons who could be construed as "victims of the machine age" (e.g., of technologically sophisticated blood products), particularly if they belonged to vulnerable populations (e.g., hemophiliacs), to whom the state might be said to owe a particular duty of care (Bell et al. 2008); and, second, the controversial legal theory—"merchandising fraud"—adopted by the trial

[5] Act Up-Paris was founded shortly before the eruption of the blood affair. The Garretta trial was a singular opportunity for the group to make itself known and establish itself (successfully) as an important player on the French AIDS scene.

[6] French law "allows victims of crimes to set in motion the criminal process by accusing a person (or person or persons unknown) of committing an offence to their prejudice, this being known as constituting themselves as *parties civiles*" (Bell et al. 2008:37). The advantages of this procedure to plaintiffs are considerable since as *partie civile* "a claimant can take advantage of the considerable investigative powers of the *juge d'instruction at the state's expense*" (Bell et al. 2008:38, emphasis added).

court (and confirmed by the court of appeals) to indict and ultimately to condemn Garretta and Allain. This theory, resting on a 1905 public health law, originated with Holleaux, one of the first lawyers to take on the hemophiliacs' case, on the grounds of its likely acceptability to the justice system (as opposed to theories of poisoning or involuntary homicide popular with many hemophiliacs).

As articulated by the courts the fraud perpetrated by Garretta and Allain had two elements, material and moral.[7] The *material* element consisted in the accused's "silence and concealment regarding the substantial qualities [of the blood products] specifically on the high risk of contamination by a deadly virus inherent in the utilization by hemophiliacs of these products sold by CNTS during the period in question [March–October 1985]."[8] The *moral* element (labeled as such by the court) was that—referring to Garretta—"he accepted the risk based on economic considerations contrary to the interests and health of hemophiliacs as evidenced by his continued sales [of contaminated products] until the stocks were exhausted." This approach to the case was by no means uniformly popular. With vocal support inside and outside the courtroom, some—not all—plaintiffs' lawyers opened the trial by attacking a theory of the case grounded on what they labeled a "crime of grocers": "Blood is merchandise??" and "The 1905 law was made for mustard, yogurt, and Perrier!" Attacks were mounted as well against a venue that did not allow a criminal trial before a jury of peers (i.e., a *cour d'assises*), and a process that failed to indict ministers in office at the time of the blood contamination. These were not treated as minor complaints either by the courts or by the French political class. The seriousness with which they were received is reflected in the fact that it took an amendment to the French Constitution allowing ministers to be indicted and brought before the courts and ten additional years of litigation to resolve them. Roux's and Netter's indictment for "non-assistance to persons in danger"—meaning that in their capacities as government officials they could have intervened to prevent the alleged danger to the health of hemophiliacs—was far less controversial although still regarded by the plaintiffs as weak given the harm inflicted.

---

[7] "Moral" comes close to what in American courts would be called *mens rea*, i.e., criminal intent.

[8] In order to come within the relevant statute of limitations, these acts must have been committed within the time frame of March 21, 1985 (three years prior to the first accepted complaint) to October 1, 1985 (the date when non-heat-treated blood products would no longer be reimbursed by the social security system).

Much to the disgust of some *parties civiles* and their legal representatives, the court threw out poisoning on the grounds that Garretta and
Allain did not *intend* to injure or kill the recipients of blood products; indeed, the plaintiffs themselves stated their purpose was medical treatment.
Establishing that hemophiliacs *were* poisoned, the court argued, was insufficient to demonstrate that poisoning was intended. In the court's judgment,
"the defendants' intention to deceive the victims is sufficiently demonstrated
by the investigation; on the other hand, nothing shows that they intended to
kill" (Greilsamer 1992:289).[9]

In their original complaints, plaintiffs targeted not only the CNTS but
also, variously, the LNS, the Comité consultative national d'éthique (CCNE),
and the Association Française des Hémophiles (AFH). The court's choice
of defendants—Garretta, Allain, Roux, and Netter—was as controversial as
the choice of legal theories. If for different reasons lawyers for both plaintiffs
and defendants agreed that the accused were "scapegoats," the real culprits
were their bosses, that is, government ministers ultimately responsible for
the conduct of public health policy. Amplified by intense media attention
and daily vocal and visual reminders from Act Up-Paris (also, of course,
heavily mediatized), the question of ministerial responsibility for blood contamination became impossible to avoid. Over that hot summer of 1992, "the
contamination drama changed its nature and turned into an affair of State"
(Hermitte 1996:435). We will return to the consequences of this shift following a more detailed account of how the actions of blood banks and public
officials were constructed and interpreted in the course of the trial.

We distinguish between (1) facts that the public prosecutor together with
lawyers on behalf of the *parties civiles* needed to establish to persuade the
three judges to convict the defendants within the terms of the 1905 law[10]and

---

[9] In French legal procedure, judgment rests far more heavily on prior investigation under the supervision of the *juge d'instruction* than (as in the United States) on argument in court. The results of
this investigation are presented by the public prosecutor in written form (known as the *réquisitoire*)
concluding in the present case with a request to the *juge d'instruction* that defendants be brought to
trial. The closest translation of *réquisitoire* is indictment. Greilsamer reproduces the text of this indictment in full.

[10] For ease of exposition, we will refer henceforth to lawyers acting on behalf of the *parties civiles*
as "prosecutors." However, it is important to understand that these lawyers are not acting on behalf of
the government, as they would in the United States, but on behalf of the claimants. A representative
of the government (*ministère public*) participates in the trial to represent the state. It was this latter
representative who signed the indictment of the four individuals accused (the *réquisitoire*) based on
information collected by an investigative arm of the state. Penalties upon conviction were fine and
imprisonment. There is no indication in Greilsamer's verbatim transcript of the court's judgment of
damages awarded to the plaintiffs. Garretta was fined 500,000 francs (approximately $92,000).

(2) the surrounding arguments and counterarguments about knowledge and responsibility. Understanding how the prosecution interpreted and applied the 1905 merchandising fraud law will be helpful when we come to compare the legal treatment of the blood affair in France with the United States. First and foremost was the controversial question of whether blood was or was not a "product." The prosecution disposed of this question in a couple of sentences, making a sharp distinction between *donated* blood, where the relation between donor and receiver (the blood bank) was wholly non-commercial (outside of commerce) and blood *derivatives*, "industrial products where the relation between manufacturer (*fabricant*) and receiver is certainly a sale, with the price established by ministerial decree" (Greilsamer 1992:292). Whole blood, in this reading of the law, is not a "product"; blood derivatives, for example, the factors injected by hemophiliacs, are a product. Second, CNCT's *responsibility* for the sale of blood products it knew to be contaminated was established by the (uncontested by the defense) fact that as manufacturer, importer, and distributor, CNCT controlled 70–80% of the French market in blood products; and (contested by the defense) by evidence of CNCT's knowledge that its products were contaminated and dangerous to their recipients. The final nail in CNTS's coffin, from the prosecution's perspective, was (again contested by the defense) evidence not only that Garretta and Allain deliberately deceived hemophiliacs (by concealing their knowledge of HIV contamination) but also that hemophiliacs were, in fact, uninformed about the quality of the products they received, specifically the mortal danger posed by these products' consumption. The faults attributed to Roux and Netter (under the "non-assistance to persons in danger" theory) were that they knew of the contamination and its dangers, had the power to intervene and prevent the distribution of contaminated products, and failed to do so. Garretta, Allain, and Roux were found guilty and Netter not guilty. Garretta was sentenced to four years in prison, with a fine of 500,000 francs, Allain was sentenced to four years with two years suspended, Roux to a four-year suspended sentence.

Surrounding these bare bones was a large scaffolding of rhetoric, vocabularies of blame and exoneration, accusations and denials of knowledge and responsibility—what Deborah Stone might characterize as "causal stories" of accident, inadvertence, or deliberate malice (Stone 1989). Threaded throughout these narratives was a powerful moral dimension centered on the identities attributed to or assumed by the accused: as physicians with a primary responsibility to their patients, grounded in the Hippocratic oath (frequently cited by the prosecution); as bureaucrats, servants of the state; or as captains of industry (principally Garretta) with an eye on the bottom line. In evaluating this rhetoric, it is important to keep in mind the bias brought by the editor (Greilsamer) to his account of the trial. Both the initial statement of the case against the defendants (*réquisitoire*) and the final judgment are official court documents; however, the description of the trial itself is a journalistic account, not a transcript. Although it includes extended quotes from participants, this account is powerfully slanted in favor of the prosecution and is thin and often mocking in its portrayal of the defense.[11]

Cohen points to the existence of a universal "cultural stock of denials" (and, we would argue, of blame) employed by individuals and governments to account for atrocities and human rights violations, illustrated in his work with examples of this process from countries across the globe (Cohen 2001:76). It is hardly surprising, then, that the rhetoric of denial and blame employed in the Paris court in the summer of 1992 not only mirrors Cohen's examples but also reappears with varying degrees of nuance in other French reports on the blood affair; the same rhetoric also appears in comparable American documents: the IOM (Institute of Medicine) report, congressional hearings, legal opinions, and the like. Both logically and in the present case— the more so because we are dealing with supposedly hard facts of medicine and science—the first set of questions concerns assertions and denials of knowledge. Much as in the pattern described by Cohen, "Among a group of defendants in the same court—Nuremburg was a notable example—accounts [varied] from innocent ignorance to arrogant self-justification" (2001:78).[12]

In its written indictment (*réquisitoire*) the *ministère public* drew upon a variety of sources—American, British, and French, scientific and administrative, public and confidential letters and reports—to establish that "by the fall of 1983, it was *known* [*on su*] that the AIDS virus was transmitted by blood and that hemophiliacs were particularly exposed"; and, further, that the defendants *knew* the virus could be inactivated by heat treatment (Greilsamer 1992:36–37). Witnesses for the defense claimed, on the contrary, that knowledge was uncertain, that heat treatment technology was unproven, that other countries did no better, and that past decisions were taken out of context

---

[11] French scientists took a very different view of the trial proceedings, as will be described below.

[12] Comparison with the Nuremberg trials may seem extreme, but it should be remembered that the crimes of Nazi Germany were experienced directly by the French people, so Holocaust analogies may have seemed more relevant to their ears than when those same analogies were employed by hemophiliacs in the United States.

and judged in the light of current knowledge, all—for better or worse—classic "denials of knowledge" (Cohen 2001). The prosecution was equally at pains to establish that hemophiliacs *did not know*, indeed that they were deliberately deceived. In moving testimony (as described by Greilsamer), the honorary president of AFH, one son dead of AIDS and another infected, stated: "Until the end, we lived with the idea that the risk of AIDS was minimal, that no hemophiliacs were infected" (Greilsamer 1992:145). The judges were persuaded, citing a meeting on May 10, 1985, where AFH adopted a motion that "there is no reason to associate AIDS and hemophilia." The judges went on, "This very positive assertion must be compared with the knowledge indisputably in possession of those in the know [*sachants*], notably Doctor Allain, who was present at this meeting." These circumstances, observed the judges, reflected the close ties between AFH and CNTS, the association's dependence on CNTS for information, and "[AFH's] total ignorance of the danger" (Greilsamer 1992:236). "The intention [of Garretta and Allain] to deceive the victims is sufficiently demonstrated" (Greilsamer 1992:289).

Attributions and denials of responsibility—for *causing* the allegedly fraudulent distribution of contaminated blood and for *resolving* the problem once identified—rested heavily on interpretations of CNTS's role as a "blood factory": its control of the market in blood products as manufacturer and distributor and as the sole French blood bank with authority to import these products (in particular, heat-treated products) from abroad. CNTS's dominant position in the market for blood products was, however, only the beginning of the story. Garretta and Allain were accused not only of engaging in deceptive practices—knowingly distributing contaminated blood products to hemophiliacs and failing to either withdraw these products or to substitute heat-treated products—but also of compounding these faults by acting for *immoral*, that is *economic*, motives.[13] The prosecution sought to establish that CNTS's struggle for preeminence in European manufacturing and distribution of blood products was the result of Garretta's overweening personal ambition and that he was responsible for the tragic consequences of his actions. The defense maintained that CNTS's actions were the outcome

---

[13] At the time of the events at issue in the trial, CNTS was in a fragile economic state and under pressure from the government to demonstrate its success in the marketplace. "Economic motives" does not refer to personal enrichment but to industrial prowess. There is ample evidence for the French government's prioritization of industrial expansion and economic competitiveness during the period leading up to the blood crisis (see, e.g., Cerny and Schain 1980).

of intense pressure from the French government in the context of its larger goals of enhancing France's competitive position both in Europe and internationally in the field of pharmaceuticals and therefore a ministerial responsibility: "The industrial policy of CNTS *set by government authorities* [*pouvoirs publics*] demanded that we prepare for the European pharmaceutical market" (Greilsamer 1992:154, emphasis added).[14] Underlying both causal stories was the theme of profane economic aspirations conflicting with (and prevailing over) the sacred duty of doctors to their patients.

Contrary to the decision-making power and responsibility attributed to them by the prosecution, Garretta and Allain (and Roux and Netter as well) consistently minimized their titles and functions and emphasized their subordinate status in the health ministerial hierarchy: "[Allain:] I am obliged to recall my very modest role in the hierarchy" (Greilsamer 1992:105). Ministers when called as witnesses pleaded lack of information and/or expertise: "The problem of heat treatment was never called to my attention," said Laurent Fabius, (Socialist) prime minister in 1985. "Since I wasn't informed, there was nothing I could do" (Greilsamer 1992:165). These "vocabularies of exoneration" are strikingly parallel to the language described by Cohen (2001) from the Nuremberg trials (see also Chapoutot 2014).

The conviction of Garretta, Allain, and Roux (as mentioned, the case against Netter was dismissed) did not end the legal process that engulfed the blood affair in France. It was not until 2003, fifteen years after the judicial system accepted the first suits brought by hemophiliacs as *parties civiles*, that the Cour de Cassation brought the process to its final conclusion by dismissing an accusation of "poisoning" brought against at least thirty public officials and physicians.[15] The complex legal maneuvers that occupied the intervening years originated in dissatisfaction with the decision of the Paris *Tribunal de Grande Instance* on two principal counts: first, the outrage of hemophiliacs at (principally Garretta's) conviction for what they regarded as a ludicrous "crime of grocers" (i.e., deception regarding the goods for sale);[16] and, second, the belief on the part of both plaintiffs and defendants

---

[14] In 1989, the Council of Europe decreed that blood products would henceforth be treated as pharmaceuticals and sold in the open European market.

[15] More specifically, the Cour de Cassation upheld the decision of the Paris Appeals Court a year earlier.

[16] Perhaps, needless to say, the outrage of hemophiliacs was a bit more complex in its origins: first, fraud pertains to goods, not people, and it was the deaths of people, hemophiliacs and their family members, that were central to their case; second, the penalty for fraud was from the plaintiffs' perspective totally insufficient.

(supported by *Le Monde* and other media outlets) that Garretta, Allain, Netter, and Roux were essentially scapegoats for the many other actors involved in the blood products business (including treating physicians) and for the three key ministers in office at the time (Fabius as prime minister; Dufoix as minister of social affairs, including health affairs; and Hervé as secretary of state for health).[17] This dissatisfaction led to the resurrection of poisoning as a legal theory and, of greater interest, to a change in the French Constitution creating a new court (La Cour de justice de la République) with the capacity to impose judgment on members of the government.[18]

The original convictions for fraud were upheld on appeal, confirming the legitimacy of the 1905 merchandising fraud law as applied to contaminated blood.[19] At the same time, the Cour de Cassation opened the door to a new and separate series of lawsuits on the grounds of poisoning. Poisoning as a legal theory had been rejected by the trial court because it required the *intention* to kill. Advocates of the poisoning theory argued that intention to kill was unnecessary; the only requisite was knowingly administrating a *potentially* lethal substance. As critics pointed out, this reading of the law would bring any doctor giving a transfusion within its scope. Nevertheless, an investigation grounded on this more liberal interpretation was initiated by the Paris court in 1994, including specifically of Garretta, much to the consternation of the Ministry of Justice since—contrary to French (as well as American) procedure—it placed him in double jeopardy. This revived investigation precipitated renewed mobilization of the media against the perceived perpetrators of a horrific crime (see, e.g., Chauveau 2011:221). Ultimately, as we noted earlier, thirty individuals, high-level civil servants, physicians, and blood bankers, were caught within the web of this new legal onslaught. Chauveau (2011:222) argues that this revived investigation grew out of a need to allow the victims of bad blood to see the full complement of individuals whom they judged responsible brought before the bar. Be that as it may, in July 2000, much to the indignation of the plaintiffs, the second case was dismissed by the Paris Court of Appeals, leaving the individuals in question free of further legal pursuit.

---

[17] Health ministry cabinet archives made clear that at least some public officials were well aware of contamination of the blood supply and its implications well before the scandal broke in 1991.

[18] Hermitte characterizes this reform as "more revolutionary than it appears." "Henceforth, any person, individual or institution, will be able to call into question the decision of a member of the government if the consequences are against the law, and the new infraction, putting a person in danger, would even allow an objection to government action in real time" (1996:437).

[19] Hermitte points out that this law was one of two pieces of legislation passed in the early 1900s with the explicit aim of protecting the public's health. At that time there was not yet a Ministry of Health, so implementation of these laws fell to the Ministry of Agriculture (1996:389–90).

This decision did not resolve—and, indeed (from a legal perspective), was quite separate from—what rapidly became in late 1992 the key question of institutional (as opposed to individual) responsibility.[20] Political and media engagement with that question, and its eventual resolution in the form of a constitutional amendment and the creation of the "Cour de justice" transformed the blood affair in France into a uniquely French "*affaire d'État*" (Hermitte 1996, Fillion 2009, Chauveau 2011). As early as December 1992, the French president, François Mitterrand, had declared in a televised address that the ministers (Fabius, Dufoix, and Hervé) should have the opportunity to demonstrate their innocence. Parliament, in part due to its political division—the three ministers were socialist, and Parliament was divided between socialists and conservatives—was unable to resolve the procedural question of how government ministers might be brought to justice. The outcome—carefully prepared and carried forward by the conservative government elected in 1993—was a constitutional amendment creating a new court specifically designed for this purpose, as noted earlier.[21] In February 1999, the three ministers were brought before this court, accused of involuntary homicide and involuntary interference with personal integrity. The cases against Fabius and Dufoix were both dismissed, while Hervé was found guilty of two counts of involuntary homicide but without penalty.

Running throughout this drawn-out legal process was a profound sense that grave moral wrongs had been done, expressed by plaintiffs and their lawyers, by public prosecutors and judges, by the media and public opinion, and by academic observers. Insofar as these wrongs had a unique "essence," it was that in their pursuit of economic, political, and/or scientific interests, governmental and commercial actors in the blood affair were indifferent to human suffering. Foremost among these malign interests (perceived as at best amoral, at worst immoral) was the pursuit of economic dominion: "It was the preference given to construction of a high performing French industry over the interests of patients that precipitated [Garretta and Allain] into [technological] delinquency" (Hermitte 1996:419).[22] The immorality of this "preference" was exacerbated in the eyes of an avid audience by the fact that the accused individuals were physicians, not only committed by their

---

[20] Multiple government and other documents had been published by 1992, virtually all of which implicated the ministers in office in 1985. "Ministers" refers to the prime minister and cabinet-level department heads (of the Ministry of Health in the present case) all of whom are political appointees.

[21] At least one French legal scholar argues that the *sole purpose* of this constitutional amendment was to prosecute ministers held responsible for the blood scandal (Beaud 1999).

[22] Hermitte uses the phrase "technological delinquency" (*délinquence technologique*) to label what she sees as specifically modern crimes arising out of flawed science and technology.

Hippocratic oath to doing "no harm" to patients but also heretofore at the pinnacle in the French pantheon of trust. These doctors' failings and those of their colleagues as portrayed in legal proceedings were experienced as a profound betrayal (Grémy 2004:195). Central to this litany of moral wrongs was what French observers saw as the dark side of scientific and technological progress. What killed hemophiliacs were the technologically sophisticated blood products they had embraced as allowing them to live a "normal" life, to "climb Mt. Blanc." Hermitte (1996:342) noted the "puzzle" of a modern technological society that is "dangerous" but at the same time supports increased expectation of life and greater security. After listing modern public health catastrophes (Tchernobyl, thalidomide, Agent Orange, Bhopal), Hermitte argued that victims of these disasters were no longer prepared to accept being treated as collateral damage in the march of progress but of a fault that should be punished. Finally, there was the immorality of the French state that abdicated its role of benevolent patriarch and betrayed its citizens, as reflected in the unconscionable ignorance and indifference of its ministers. The governors failed to govern.

The moral outrage we have described is pervasive not only in French popular literature on the blood affair but also in the scholarly writing on which we have drawn both for the narrative of this event and for the meanings attributed to it. An alternative perspective is suggested by an article in the American journal *Science* that appeared on January 28, 1994, following the conviction of Garretta, Allain, and Roux and the failure of their appeal. The article, datelined Paris and headlined, "French AIDS Scandal," described a letter to President François Mitterrand from "nearly 100 researchers" asking that these "doctors" be pardoned on the grounds that "the court did not allow expert scientific testimony about the decisions that were made" (p. 461). The letter was drafted by prominent French scientists Jean-Claude Gluckmann and Nobel laureate Françoise Barré-Sinousi. The letter stated that the four doctors "were victims of 'trial by the media, where sensationalism dominated to the detriment of accuracy, and passionate debate took the place of objective facts'" (p. 461). Similar claims were made in a second letter sent to Mitterrand signed by thirty-two Nobel laureates asking a pardon for Allain alone, a campaign organized by Cambridge University molecular biologist Max Perutz. These letters were dismissed by France's minister of health—"Justice has been done. Those voices that are expressing themselves today should have expressed themselves earlier"—and were received with anger by the French public, according to *Science*. There is no evidence that these letters had any impact on the course of events. The pursuit of "justice" continued.

United States

"Culpable conduct with impunity."[23] There was no comparable show trial or constitutional reckoning in the United States. American courts were, in fact, extraordinarily unfriendly to plaintiffs in blood cases, whether they were infected by transfusion or through blood products. In the course of his opinion dated March 16, 1995, on a motion to dismiss a class action suit brought by hemophiliacs against a blood manufacturer, Judge Richard Posner observed that as of that date some 300 cases had been filed by hemophiliacs and/or their next of kin. Thirteen of those cases had been tried in various courts around the country "and the defendants have won twelve of them" (*In the Matter of Rhone-Poulenc Rorer* 1995). Whether plaintiffs sued blood banks, manufacturers of blood products, or the FDA, and whether their theory of liability was fraud and misrepresentation (nearest to the winning French "crime of grocers"), breach of warranty, or strict liability, they lost. Poisoning and involuntary homicide were never considered. The only winning theory was negligence, successful in a single isolated case, *Quintana vs. United Blood Services*. The most significant obstacles confronting the plaintiffs in United States' courts were the "blood shield" statutes in effect in all but three states and the District of Columbia. In a supreme irony, the legal theory that was successful in France—the "crime of grocers"—was precluded in the United States. The language of the applicable Colorado statute, essentially identical to the other forty-seven states is unambiguous:

> The donation, whether for or without valuable consideration, the acquisition, preparation, transplantation, injection, or transfusion of any ... blood, or component thereof for or to a human being is the performance of a medical service and does not, in any way, constitute a sale. No ... blood bank who donates, obtains, ... injects, transfuses, or otherwise transfers, from one or more human beings, living or dead, to another living human being for the purpose of therapy or transplantation needed by him for his health

[23] We have appropriated this title from a law journal article with the same name by Linda M. Dorney, "Culpable Conduct with Impunity: The Blood Industry and the FDA's Responsibility for the Spread of AIDS Through Blood Products," 3 *J. Pharmacy & L.* 129 (1994).

or welfare shall be liable for any damages of any kind or description directly or indirectly caused by or resulting from any such activity; *except that each such person or entity remains liable for his or its own negligence or willful misconduct.*" (*Quintana v. United Blood Services* 1991, emphasis in original)

State legislatures have justified this and comparable statutes on the grounds of "public health and welfare" and the desire to promote an adequate blood supply; the *Quintana* court took a more cynical view: "The statute defines blood related activities as a medical service solely to ensure the preclusion of claims which might arise if such activities are characterized as a commercial sale of a product" (*Quintana* 1991:5). In language rare among state courts that ruled on these cases, this court recognized that the characterization of blood transactions as a "service" was a fiction designed to protect suppliers. That the blood industry operates, in fact, as an extremely profitable regime of buyers and sellers has been well documented (Rock 1986, Gaul 1989b, Starr [1998] 2002).

The effect of blood shield laws was to make "negligence or willful misconduct" on the part of the blood bank or manufacturer the only legal theory on which Americans infected with HIV from blood or blood products could hope to prevail.[24] The "negligence" of which defendants were accused in *Quintana* and other blood cases was "failing properly to screen blood donors and ... failing to implement testing procedures that would have indicated the presence of AIDS in the donated blood that plaintiff had received" (*Quintana* 1991:3). The reasoning of the appeals court in the *Quintana* case illustrates both how "knowledge" about blood contamination was understood and deployed in an American court *relatively* friendly to the HIV-infected plaintiff and the roadblocks that the plaintiff confronted.

"Negligence" in common law is defined as "failure to exercise the care toward others which a reasonable or prudent person would do in the circumstances or taking action which such a reasonable person would not" (dictionary.law.com, accessed 3/8/21). In determining what a "reasonable or prudent" blood bank or blood products manufacturer should

---

[24] The FDA is protected from lawsuits by a complex set of regulations, including that "[decisions] regarding how to protect the nation's blood supply and blood recipients from the AIDS threat are [discretionary, that is] decisions that are susceptible to policy analysis; they require the decision-maker to balance the degree of risk against the social, economic, and political costs of prevention." The key word in this language is "discretionary" (*C.R.S. v. United States*, 820 F. Supp. 449 (D. Minn. 1993); cited in Dorney 1994:163). Only if its employee violated a binding rule or regulation will a government agency be held accountable.

have done "in the circumstances," the majority of American courts relied on the prevailing industry custom or practice at the time in question; the *Quintana* court rejected this standard observing that "there was undisputed evidence at trial . . . that the AABB [American Association of Blood Bank] recommendations and FDA regulations represented only *minimum* standards and that these standards differed as between whole blood and plasma banks" (*Quintana* 1991:7, emphasis in original). The *Quintana* court held that the plaintiff should have the opportunity to prove through expert testimony that the entire blood industry's customs and practices were negligent.

Central to establishing negligence were much the same questions about the state of medical/scientific knowledge in the period 1980–1985 that confronted the Garretta court and, indeed, confronted commentators in both countries who sought (or sought to avoid) accountability to victims of HIV-blood contamination. The questions—explicit or implicit—addressed in the factual determinations of the Garretta as well as the American courts went well beyond the classic "who knew what, when" questions about HIV transmission through the blood supply, the dangers to transfusion recipients and hemophiliacs, and alternative preventive measures. These questions included not only who knew what and when but also what knowledge was relevant, whose knowledge counted, whose knowledge was heard or discounted, what were the critical time periods, and who could be trusted to decide these questions. None of the answers were self-evident. They were contingent on the sympathies and interests (personal, political, economic, industrial) of the person or agency to whom the questions were directed.[25]

A critical difference between the Garretta court and American courts that confronted these questions at any time prior to the publication of the IOM report in 1995 was the presence (in the French case) and absence (in the American case) of a prior widely recognized authoritative narrative of the "facts." The Lucas report "Transfusion and AIDS in 1985: Chronology of Facts and Decisions Concerning Hemophiliacs" was published in September 1991. Michel Lucas was the director of IGAS, the French state's investigative arm for "social affairs." The report was requested in June 1991 by Jean-Louis Bianco and Bruno Durieux in their official capacities as, respectively, minister of social affairs and integration and minister of health, for the purpose

---

[25] Most American courts never reached these substantive questions, dismissing blood cases on a variety of procedural grounds.

of "establishing in a precise and exhaustive manner the reality and chronology of facts and decisions with regard to blood transfusion as it affects hemophiliacs." In this context the legitimacy and authority of the Lucas report was unquestioned; it was cited (selectively) throughout the indictment (*réquisitoire*) from the Ministry of Justice that grounded the trial of Garretta, Allain, Roux, and Netter.[26]

There was no comparably authoritative report of the "facts" on which American courts might rely before the publication in 1995 of the IOM's report "HIV and the Blood Supply: A Study of Crisis Decision Making" (also, like the Lucas report, focused on hemophiliacs).[27] Judges in earlier cases wrote their own narratives and often disagreed, as exemplified by the *Quintana* court's objection to the use of the defendant blood bank's evidence to determine the "standard of care." Among plaintiffs' many obstacles in these cases were the decisions of several federal appeals courts that precluded the deposition of expert witnesses from government agencies (e.g., the CDC) who were most familiar with *what* was known in the early days of the HIV-blood affair, *when* it was known, and *who* knew it. After resigning from the CDC, Donald Francis, who had been director of the CDC's AIDS Laboratory, testified in the second *Quintana* trial to devastating effect. Referring to the actions of blood bankers in the early 1980s, he said: "It was something like standing at a bend in a train track, you hear the whistle, the signal is blinking, the track is beginning to shake and they're saying, 'there's no train coming.'"[28]

Whether French or American, advocates for the victims of toxic blood argued that knowledge came early, was certain, and was actionable, and the accused—blood banks, manufacturers, and some government officials—argued that knowledge was late, uncertain, and not actionable. Each accused the other of distorting history to suit their interests of the moment.

---

[26] Over twenty years later, in Nathanson's first interview with a French cabinet official regarding the blood affair, the only document he recommended to her was the Lucas report. We will discuss this report in more detail in Chapter 8 in the context of other French reports on the blood affair as well as the IOM report.

[27] Once the IOM report was published, political and judicial bodies that addressed questions regarding the blood supply referred to it as "the" authoritative source.

[28] Sue Lindsay, "Official: Blood Test Plea Ignored U.S. Researcher Pushed for AIDS Screening in 1983, but Blood Banks Refused Despite Spread of Disease, Jury Told," *Rocky Mountain News*, July 18, 1992, 30. The Quintanas prevailed in this case and were awarded $8 million in damages, but by that time Susie Quintana had died.

7

The Quest for Compensation

Whether and how generously governments—as opposed to private
individuals or institutions—compensate injuries to their citizens (and/
or injuries that occur within their territorial boundaries) is contingent on
cross-nationally variable assumptions about the scope of government responsibility, as well as on short-term political considerations. Within these
constraints, advocates for one or another solution create causal stories—
competing portrayals of "facts" and of the moral implications of those facts
(Gusfield 1981, Stone 1989). In the case of HIV-contaminated blood, these
stories were prefigured in the analogies political actors used to make their
case: a holocaust, a terrorist attack, a natural disaster (e.g., earthquake, hurricane, or flood) or, rather less dramatically, vaccine-related injuries. Each
of these analogies contained underlying assumptions—or images—of the
causal chain that produced the harm in question; specifically, assumptions
about the locations of responsibility for causing—and redressing—the bad
outcome. These analogies were offered by political actors in the course of
public hearings in France and in the United States as precedents for government compensation of persons who acquired HIV/AIDS from toxic blood.
Holocaust and terrorism invoked faceless evildoers as ultimately responsible,
while disaster was equivalent to accident, where no identifiable human motive was at work: an act of God. Compensation for vaccine-related injuries
was a recent precedent in both countries.

Militant hemophiliacs in France along with their allies in the media
constructed precisely targeted causal chains, precipitating political crisis,
and forcing government action to generously compensate persons who
contracted HIV from contaminated blood and blood products (i.e., by transfusion or injection). Militants in the United States did the same, but in the absence of sustained media and elite political support and with little visibility,
their efforts took longer, the results were not so generous, and transfusion-
infected persons were excluded. From the perspective of political authorities

The Social Production of Crisis. Constance A. Nathanson and Henri Bergeron, Oxford University Press.
© Oxford University Press 2023. DOI: 10.1093/oso/9780197682487.003.0007

in the United States, the disaster metaphor had the double advantage of designating hemophiliacs as innocent victims and of conflating compensation with "disaster relief," an accepted government function.[1] Invoking government responsibility through the conflation of HIV contamination with natural disaster rather than with government malfeasance was, in the United States, the only politically feasible route to compensation.

An alternative analogy is between blood and other potentially dangerous products: alcohol, tobacco, cocaine, guns. The chain of causation in each case is nearly identical—substance-user-seller-manufacturer-raw materials supplier-regulator—and applies equally well to blood and blood products.[2] Each element in the chain has both an empirical and a moral status: empirically, smoking causes lung cancer; morally, lung cancer has been blamed on the irresponsible smoker (either for smoking herself or for endangering others); occasionally, the vendor; most often the manufacturer; sometimes the government regulator. Empirically—to spell out the parallel with blood—HIV/AIDS is caused by transmission of bodily fluids (including blood) that carry the human immunodeficiency virus from one person to another. Morally, responsibility and blame for HIV/blood infection have been attached at every point in the causal chain, from hemophiliacs and transfusees themselves, to the doctors that treated them, to the blood banks and fractionators that purveyed the tainted blood, to the regulators that failed to regulate, to the state that failed at every level, from warning blood users to governing the blood system.

France

At the end of December 1991, the French Parliament passed a law that included (among an assortment of other unrelated provisions), Article 47, to compensate "victims of injury resulting from HIV contamination caused by blood transfusion or injection of blood products occurring on the territory of

---

[1] Stone describes political actors seeking government action as pushing causal stories in the direction of willful and intentional behavior. And this was certainly true of militant actors in both countries. This analysis suggests the further point that weaving of causal stories is highly contingent on political opportunity structures that may vary from one country to another.

[2] We are powerfully indebted to Deborah Stone whose work led us to realize the aptness of the analogy between other dangerous products and human blood (Stone 1989). We have slightly adapted the causal chain she proposes by adding (government) regulators.

the French Republic."[3] Eligibility for compensation encompassed transfusees as well as hemophiliacs (and their legal beneficiaries) from the date of HIV infection.[4] It was generous, its procedures were simple and straightforward (limited to showing infection and the use of blood or blood products) and, by all accounts, quick and efficient (Hermitte 1996:325). Notably, it did not require that applicants to the compensation fund drop lawsuits against transfusion centers or other defendants that they may have had underway (as had a previous—highly discredited—version).

The 1991 law was passed by the French Parliament in the depth of political crisis. In June 1991, shortly after the publication of Casteret's inflammatory article in *l'Événement du jeudi*, the minister of health had told the National Assembly that "irrespective of the actions in court now underway . . . the exceptional character of the situation requires us to put in place a rapid and just compensation system, grounded in *solidarité*" (Hermitte 1996:323). Evoking "solidarity" allowed the minister to side-step questions of responsibility. Compensation would be grounded in French citizens' mutual obligation to support one another in time of need—a quintessential act of *solidarité*— not in recognition of government responsibility for its failure to protect the blood supply.

On November 10, 1991, the compensation fund was endorsed by the president of the republic, François Mitterrand. This rapid action is testimony to the opportunity created by an immediate political crisis but obscures the less visible social process of crisis production carried out over the preceding five years by hemophiliacs, transfusees, and their allies in Parliament and the media. Principal actors in this drama included officials in the health ministry, members of Parliament, hemophiliacs and transfusees, and journalists, each with their own causal stories. Our sources for these actors' narratives include Health Ministry cabinet archives, parliamentary reports and debates, newspaper archives, and a wide range of secondary sources.[5]

In the spring of 1987, the Association Française des Hémophiles (AFH) approached the Ministry of Health—deferentially and without

---

[3] *LOI no 91-1406 du 31 décembre 1991 portant diverses dispositions d'ordre social.*

[4] Who should be covered by the law was a point of contention (e.g., why not people with hepatitis?), and additional groups were added in later years.

[5] The most important of these secondary sources are the postdoctoral thesis of Sophie Chauveau, who had full access to archives of the DGS and Emmanuelle Fillion's book-length treatment of hemophiliacs' experience of HIV/AIDS, much of it drawn from the archives of the AFH and Fillion's interviews with AFH representatives during the period in question. Marie-Angèle Hermitte's *Le Sang et le Droit (Blood and Law)* is an in-depth legal appreciation of the French blood affair, and among the earliest (1996) scholarly accounts.

publicity—asking for financial relief for families of hemophiliacs who had lost fathers and sons to AIDS. The scope of loss and of infection was by that date highly visible within this small and tightly knit community; the president of the AFH was himself infected (and died in 1988). Compensation was floated in Parliament that fall, and the AFH renewed its lobbying of the Health Ministry. These efforts—continued over the next two years—met with substantial resistance from the Ministry of Health and only bore fruit under the pressure of events outside the power of the government to manage or control.[6] Earlier we described the blood affair as a drama in two acts. In the French version of this drama, Act II has two scenes: before Casteret ("the theatre is dimly lit"), and after Casteret ("the lights go up"). Compensation during Scene 1 was negotiated internally and to no one's satisfaction; the second round of negotiations (Scene 2) played out in the public eye.

Central to these negotiations were causal stories advanced in parallel by the multiple actors in this drama, shifting over time, less on the basis of new information than of changing political opportunities, strategic alliances, and fields of power.[7] As we noted earlier, the AFH in its early approaches to the government was very clear in its reluctance to cast blame on doctors and transfusion centers "with whom [hemophiliacs] must live their entire lives" (Hermitte 1996:349). In a trope that reappeared frequently in French accounts of the blood crisis, the AFH framed the desired relief as "a gesture of solidarity for *victims of technical progress*, not as compensation for damages" (Fillion 2009:145, emphasis added).[8] The government (or at least its administrative services) saw the proposed relief somewhat differently, as we have seen, arguing that "compensation" set a bad precedent in its implication of government responsibility (FNA, Box 910611-1[CAB 506], January 14, 1988).[9]

---

[6] It is important to remind the reader that 1986–1988 was the period of "cohabitation" when France had a Socialist president (Mitterrand), but the government was in the hands of conservatives under Jacques Chirac as prime minister. In 1987 through mid-May 1988, when Socialists returned to power and Claude Evin took over the health ministry, the minister was Michele Barzach.

[7] Although we cannot state it with absolute certainty, every evidence indicates that the facts that became central to this drama—delayed approval of HIV testing and delayed withdrawal of non-heat-treated blood products from the market—were in possession of the principal actors certainly from 1987 and very possibly 1986.

[8] This idea had no traction in the United States. When technical progress comes up, it is invariably in a context where hemophiliacs (a) should be grateful for it, (b) embraced it to their detriment, (c) can look forward to it solving their problems in the future.

[9] As in Chapter 4, all of the quotes from and references to cabinet documents in this chapter are from Box 910611-1, CAB 506 (cabinet of health minister, Claude Evin), located in the French National Archives (FNA). In subsequent references, we follow the same procedure and abbreviate reference to those materials as "FNA" followed by the date.

Newspapers clippings included in a folder from the cabinet archives (labeled Hemophilia/AIDS/Solidarity Fund for Persons Contaminated with the AIDS Virus from Blood Transfusion) point to the difficulty confronted by this cabinet in deflecting government responsibility: from *Le Monde*, both dated February 22, 1988, "Several Thousand Transfused Contaminated/ A Solidarity Fund for AIDS"; and "This Situation, Still Little Known to the Public, Appears Particularly Difficult for the *Government* to Manage." This same article states that "associations that defend the rights of hemophiliacs and the multiply transfused [a reference to Garvanoff's association of hemophiliac militants] do not conceal their dissatisfaction with the attention [to this affair] paid by the *government*" (emphases added). Implied, if not explicit, in these observations by *Le Monde*'s senior medical journalist was that political responsibility for the blood affair belonged to the government, however much the government might wish to disown it.[10]

From 1988 through 1991, a succession of ministerial cabinets were battered both publicly and privately by an escalating drumbeat of alternative narratives driven by a growing cast that rapidly came to include increasingly well-organized, coordinated, and media-savvy associations of "victims" and media elites eager to hear their stories. In public the cabinets stuck stubbornly to their narrative that "the immense majority of the scientific and medical community did not [in 1985 and before] have the knowledge required to confront the danger," that attribution of responsibility was up to the judiciary, and that the proposed *fonds de solidarité* (compensation) was entirely exceptional, equivalent to a recently adopted law to compensate victims of terrorism, and not a precedent (Sénat 1991c:5379 [statement of Jean-Louis Bianco]).[11] Cabinet archives make clear that internally and in private, this narrative of medical ignorance and impossibility had broken down long before Bianco's speech to Parliament in late 1991.

As we described in Chapter 3, the assault by militant hemophiliacs—documented in the Evin cabinet archives—began almost immediately after the Socialist government returned to power in the spring of 1988.[12]

---

[10] Note that the *Le Monde* article was published early in 1988, three years before the Casteret article in l'*Événement du jeudi*.

[11] We suggested earlier that mass murder models (e.g., terrorism, holocaust) had more historical resonance in France than in the United States.

[12] A ministry in France has two arms, the "administration"—the more or less permanent civil service—and the cabinet. The ministerial cabinet is a uniquely French institution; its members are handpicked by and serve at the pleasure of their minister. The minister is a political appointee who—along with her cabinet—comes and goes with the fortunes of the government in power. The interests

Following up his initial May 5, 1988, letter to Evin stating that "the scandal [of hemophiliacs] has been deliberately smothered" by the prior government, Garvanoff wrote a month later to the new prime minister pointing the finger both at Garretta's Centre National de Transfusion Sanguine (CNTS) and at the AFH ("their language is very different from ours") and calling particular attention to the 1985 "delay" in taking non-heat-treated blood products off the market.[13] This missive was forwarded by the prime minister's cabinet officials to their counterparts in the Evin cabinet with a request to please provide a response "without delay."[14]

The AFH had been meeting quietly and discreetly with the Conservative health minister (Barzach) since the spring of 1987. However urgent Garvanoff's pleas, the immediate response of the Evin cabinet was hardly welcoming. The cabinet official assigned to reply to the prime minister's request did answer "without delay" (within 48 hours) that these new actors on the scene were to be treated as illegitimate upstarts. The only legitimate interlocutor was the AFH. The remainder of this internal cabinet memo, dated June 7, was a review of what its author labeled "obstacles to compensation," principally the implied engagement of responsibility by the state. Notably, the cabinet official tied the threat of state (and CNTS) engagement to the same events cited by Garvanoff—the delay in implementing heat treatment of blood products intended for hemophiliacs, making clear that this narrative was on the table in private among members of the government well before it emerged on the public stage. Alluding to the chaotic legal climate—lawsuits already brought and on the horizon with unpredictable outcomes—the author recommended that compensation be "studied," the implication being that compensation would deflect action in the courts. In the meantime, the AFH should be welcomed enthusiastically by the minister, but not until

of the cabinet "are those of the minister, which also means that [the cabinet] is deeply concerned with the general policies [and politics] of the government of the day" (Suleiman 1974:211). The interests of the "administration" are framed as internal and "technical," those of the cabinet as external and political, attuned to and reflecting any political winds that might affect "their" minister.

[13] There was, indeed, a period of three months between the government's announcement on August 1, 1985, that non-heat-treated products would no longer be reimbursed by the health care system and October 1, when this policy went into effect. This period was central to hemophiliacs', transfusees', and the media case against the government. We have put "delay" in quotes to signal that contest.

[14] The Evin cabinet was under enormous political pressure to come forward with a major response to the larger AIDS epidemic. The cabinet was totally absorbed by this effort and regarded hemophiliacs as a relatively minor ripple in this much larger ocean (Evin cabinet official, author interview, November 4, 2010).

the "*dossier*" was complete.[15] This memo was a classic example of French cabinet-speak as described by Suleiman (1974:316ff.): civil society groups were "consulted" only if they were perceived as "legitimate" and only on the cabinet's terms; policies were "explained" to interested outside groups once those policies had been decided internally.

As pressure mounted—both internally from other ministries and Parliament and externally, not only from AFH and the press but also from the CNTS and insurance companies—the façade that the Health Ministry was not responsible for what a few media outlets had already framed as a health debacle became increasingly difficult to sustain. The intensity of this pressure was reflected in almost daily memos written by the responsible cabinet official in the early months of 1989. In sometimes poignant detail, he recorded demands for action, threats of lawsuits and public exposure, and cracks in the comfortable narrative of expert incapacity. "Now that the facts are becoming known to the public and, in particular, to the victims, the solidarity of those in charge in concealing [those facts] splinters. . . . [*Le Monde*] is playing on these mutual recriminations" (FNA, March 30, 1989). The anguish and frustration of this official (whom we will call Mr. X) were patent. Labeling his dossier as "explosive" and his memo "urgent and confidential," Mr. X wrote to his minister, "it is increasingly evident that massive infection from blood transfusion continued even after blood testing became obligatory on August 1, 1985, with full knowledge of the parties responsible." Mr. X went on to state that "it was known with certainty by 1983 that the AIDS virus was transmitted by blood donation," that heat-treated American blood products available by 1985 were "deliberately" rejected to protect CNTS's monopoly, and that blood collection had continued in "risky populations" (i.e., in prisons). "Today, *everyone turns to the State* and, in particular, to the Minister, to manage a dramatic problem: early death of thousands infected at a time when many believe their deaths could have been prevented" (FNA, March 30, 1989, emphasis added). What was, in the United States, framed as a "complex" problem with plenty of blame to go around, was rapidly simplified in France to a problem for the state.

In repeated memos that circulated within the cabinet and between the cabinet and the Direction Générale de la Santé (DGS) during this period, officials described their efforts to restrain the AFH from going public and/

---

[15] It is unclear to what precise dossier the author refers, most probably not to compensation but to a proposed new program for medical and social care for hemophiliacs.

or to court, to placate the CNTS (in the person of Garretta), and to stave off the press, efforts tied directly to what became the increasingly "urgent" matter of a "solidarity fund" (phrasing adopted to avoid the word "compensation"): "The longer we wait, the more difficult this problem will be to manage" (FNA, January 23, 1989). Fraught negotiations culminated in an agreement signed in early July 1989, by the state, transfusion centers, their insurers, and the AFH.[16] The agreement applied only to hemophiliacs (as opposed to the much larger population of individuals infected through blood transfusion). It created two funds: one private funded by the insurers that allocated the equivalent of $20,000 to anyone who was sero-positive, and a second one funded by the state that was somewhat more generous, directed to persons with AIDS, their widowed spouses, and children. These funds were framed as charitable acts. There was no acknowledgment of responsibility on the part of transfusion centers or the state, and beneficiaries of the private fund were required to confirm in writing they would not bring suit against these centers or their insurers.

The appearance of consensus around this agreement almost immediately fell apart. The key actors in this drama—principally hemophiliacs but quickly joined by victims of toxic blood transfusion—leaked its essential elements into the public sphere, laying the groundwork for a crisis that left the political establishment no option but (slowly and, at first grudgingly) to acknowledge responsibility and mount a robust response. The AFH benefited from the pressure exerted by its radical flank, the ADP, and both benefited from the attentive ear of the press, principally the medical journalists of *Le Monde*. On January 23, 1989, the responsible cabinet official had warned his minister (Evin) that *Le Monde* had the whole story (*tout un dossier sous le coude*) and was being restrained with difficulty. On April 28, a few days after Evin announced that a "*fonds de solidarité*" (the protocol described above) would be created, *Le Monde* published the "dossier" in a two-page spread under the headline, "AIDS: The Scandal of Hemophiliacs."

In a sidebar under the heading, "A Lack of Judgment," the article quoted at length from a letter AFH had sent Evin the previous August (1988) calling attention in particular to the 1985 decision to delay withdrawal from circulation of blood products known to be HIV contaminated until existing stocks were exhausted. Another sidebar headlined "The Price of Fault," quoted Jean

---

[16] This agreement was negotiated internally within the governments' relevant ministries. Parliament was not involved.

Peron Garvanoff, the head of ADP, on the *fonds*: "The issue for us, certainly, is to obtain compensation, but also and above all to denounce the errors" (i.e., to assign responsibility). In the same space, Garvanoff attacked the AFH for its "policy of discretion" and cozy relations with the transfusion establishment. Curiously, this article made few ripples at the time it was published; nevertheless, it clearly anticipated the political scandal that was to come and framed the issues in the exact terms central to the crisis when it did erupt two years later: "Who was responsible? Who must pay?" (Nau 1989). Key to understanding how this crisis was socially produced are this reporter's close relationships with leaders of the hemophiliac community (both the "discrete" AFH and its radical flank), on which he clearly relied.

On November 17, 1989, the minister of health again insisted publicly (in a statement prepared by the health administration, always more conservative than the politically attuned cabinet) that before 1985, it was "scientifically impossible" to prevent HIV-blood contamination, referring both to experts at the time and to an "expert" letter published a few days earlier in *Le Monde* (a letter that had been solicited by the health ministry). It was signed by four mandarins of the transfusion service plus the head of the French Association of Blood Donors stating that prior to a conference held in Atlanta in April 1985 it was impossible to know whether heat treatment was safe and effective. The AFH, under increasing pressure from the ADP and with the knowledge that a Paris court had awarded a victim of transfusion AIDS over twenty times the compensation available from the *fonds*, was not impressed. On February 22, 1990, in a meeting at the Ministry of Health characterized by the cognizant cabinet official as a "high stakes negotiation," the AFH took the position that their only legitimate interlocutor was the state—"not insurance companies!"—that the amount of compensation they were offered was not nearly sufficient, and that although reluctant to go to court, they had no alternative.

In the meantime, pointed questions were being asked in Parliament, and in February 1990 *Le Monde* announced the formation of a new association (Association des Transfusées [ADT]) for individuals infected through blood transfusion. The latter were described by the ADT's spokesperson (in implicit contrast to hemophiliacs), as "isolated across France without any point in common except their suffering and their misery" and demanded compensation on the model of victims of terrorism (Nau 1990). In April 1990, a member of the French Senate, Claude Huriet, tabled a *"proposition de loi"* based on the premises that the Evin protocol was inadequate, that the French state was entirely responsible for regulation of the transfusion system, and that hemophiliacs should be compensated on the model of compensation for vaccination injuries.[17] Although questions about compensation for persons infected with HIV through transfusion had been raised earlier in Parliament and the press, ADT was the first organized group to embrace compensation for the transfused as its central purpose. ADT's president was an extremely well-connected former senator and minister, a "friend" of Mitterrand, who had no hesitation in threatening direct action (e.g., boycotts of blood dona-tion, public demonstrations, a "flood" of lawsuits) to get compensation for his association's members. Nor was he in any doubt that "the government is responsible and must acknowledge [its responsibility]" (Nothias 1991b).

Faced with a rapidly unfolding public scandal and a network of highly mobilized civil society actors, the French government was forced to abandon its much maligned Evin protocol. Legislation creating a far more generous compensation package that covered transfusees as well as hemophiliacs was proposed and passed on December 31, 1991, as described in the opening paragraph of this section. This was still, however, a *fonds de solidarité*, not—insisted the minister of health (Bianco)—an acknowledgment of govern-ment responsibility. The question of responsibility and the implications of one or another interpretation of and answer to this question were heatedly discussed in the course of parliamentary debate. Controversy—and overt politicization—of the compensation bill were muted only by conservative members' desire to avoid any opening for the attribution of strict liability (re-sponsibility without fault) to physicians for medical errors, a pattern scorn-fully identified as an "American peculiarity." A resolution in favor not so much of acknowledging government responsibility as no longer contesting it took a change of ministry leadership (from Bianco to Bernard Kouchner).[18] Debate on the question of how to allocate responsibility and compensate victims not only of contaminated blood but also of medical errors more broadly continued in France over the next fifteen years, culminating in a law passed on March 4, 2002, creating a mechanism of compensation for victims of medical errors with or without "responsibility" (Cour des comptes 2017).

[17] A *"proposition de loi"* is a law proposed by a member of Parliament. Laws proposed by the gov-ernment are labeled *"projets de loi."*
[18] Under Kouchner, all persons who could document that they were HIV positive and had either injected blood products or were transfused were compensated irrespective of the dates when infec-tion occurred. Further, the state would no longer contest suits brought by potential beneficiaries against the fund itself (e.g., pursuant to rejection of their application). As noted by an official of the DGS in deploring this move, it amounted to an acknowledgment of responsibility.

Apart from the letter to *Le Monde* cited above and scattered references to Garretta (who was as eager as the AFH for the state to assume responsibility for compensation), there is little evidence in the cabinet archives, parliamentary debates, or the media of pushback against compensation (however generous) on the part of either blood bankers or the well-organized French Federation of Blood Donors.[19] Once the scandal broke, these actors were quickly discredited: whatever counterarguments or alternative narratives they may have wished to propose found little reception in the media or elsewhere.[20] Their only available venue was the courts where they were on trial, and by the time the trial of Garretta and Jean-Pierre Allain (CNTS medical director) was underway in the summer of 1992, the reputation of French blood bankers had been thoroughly destroyed.

United States

President Clinton signed the Ricky Ray Hemophilia Relief Fund Act into law on November 12, 1998. It took two additional years and aggressive lobbying by hemophiliacs and their allies for the Relief Fund to be funded through the congressional appropriations process, some eight years after the similar, but far more generous and inclusive, law was passed and funded in France. Among the most consequential difference between the two laws was the Ricky Ray Act's omission of individuals infected by transfusion: "compensation" was confined to hemophiliacs.[21] Second, eligibility for compensation under

---

[19] Pushback was limited to ethicists and a few parliamentarians concerned about "exclusion" from compensation of other victims seen as equally deserving. We address this question later in the chapter.

[20] The extent of discreditation is strikingly reflected in the article cited in the previous chapter relatively sympathetic to France's blood bankers published in *Science* on January 28, 1994. Headlined, "Letters Provoke Unintended Response," the article states: "When nearly 100 researchers wrote last week to President François Mitterrand asking him to pardon the four doctors convicted for their role in France's HIV-contaminated blood scandal, they could not have anticipated the angry public reaction their letter touched off. Two of the convicted physicians . . . are currently in prison, and from the tenor of French press coverage, much of the public wants them to stay there." (Balter 1994:461). The reporter cites a similar letter to Mitterrand signed by "12 Nobel laureates and six other well-known scientists." This "campaign" was organized by a Nobel laureate who is quoted as stating, "From the evidence [I have seen], I became convinced that Allain [one of the four doctors] is innocent." Notable is both the sympathetic treatment of these doctors that an American scientific audience was shown and the total dismissal of their case by a French audience. As noted earlier, the article quotes Simone Veil, French minister of health in 1994 (in a now conservative government): "Justice has been done. The voices that are expressing themselves today should have expressed themselves earlier."

[21] Use of the word "compensation" in connection with the Ricky Ray Act was taboo according to Resnik's respondents. We will return to this point below.

the Ricky Ray Act was limited to individuals (or surviving spouses, children, or parents in that order) infected between July 1, 1982, and December 31, 1987. The French law required only the demonstration of HIV infection together with the use of blood or blood products irrespective of dates. Third, not only were payments from the Ricky Ray Fund deferred by the time it took to get the law funded, but they were also—in relative terms—stingy, limited to $100,000 per person irrespective of individual economic, social, and medical circumstances.[22] Further, much of the language in the Ricky Ray Act was devoted to ensuring that payments under the fund would not either render the recipients ineligible for means-tested benefits (Medicaid, Social Security) or be swallowed up by demands from insurance companies or other third parties. And finally, in contrast not only to the French bill but also to an earlier version of the Ricky Ray bill that failed to pass, the Ricky Ray Hemophilia Relief Fund Act of 1998 contained an explicit disavowal of government responsibility. Under the heading "Humanitarian Nature of Payment," the legislation states:

This Act does not create or admit any claim of or on behalf of the individual against the United States or against any officer, employee, or agent thereof acting within the scope of employment or agency that relate to an HIV infection arising from treatment with antihemophilic factor, at any time during the period beginning on July 1, 1982, and ending on December 31, 1987. A payment under this Act shall, however, when accepted by or on behalf of the individual, be in full satisfaction of all such claims by or on behalf of that individual.[23]

[22] The total appropriation for Ricky Ray, covering (in principle) between 8,000–10,000 persons, was approximately $900 million. The estimated expenditure for around 11,000 French cases (hemophiliacs and transfusees) was $1.2–1.4 billion (Steffen 1999:116), slightly over 1.5 times the appropriation for Ricky Ray. The logic behind French payouts was similar to that in an American torts case, taking account of economic loss as well as pain and suffering and, hence, varying from person to person.

[23] The conditions under which an individual or other entity may bring suit against the U.S. government are murky at best. Testimony in the first hearing on the Ricky Ray bill argued that under the Federal Tort Claims Act "the United States is not liable for its conduct in regulating or in failing to regulate private conduct that causes injuries" and, consequently, is immunized "from tort liability [for] the decisions of regulatory agencies concerning the measures taken, or the measures not taken, to respond to the incidence of the HIV virus in the nation's blood supply in the 1980s" (U.S. House of Representatives 1996:168). This rhetoric did not prevent later commentators from interpreting the Ricky Ray Act as an acknowledgment of government responsibility for the plight of hemophiliacs.

Six months after Ricky Ray bill was first introduced in February 1995, an editorial writer for the *Philadelphia Inquirer* called his readers attention to a "worthy, but little noticed bill dealing with the plight of AIDS-infected hemophiliacs . . . [a bill] which has received virtually no public attention, but surely warrants it" (Klein 1995: A9). The *Philadelphia Inquirer* was, in fact, the *only* major print newspaper in the United States to give "the plight of hemophiliacs" sustained news (as well as editorial) coverage extending from the mid-1980s through 2000. Bayer describes the "studied silence" on the bill of the Clinton administration (a silence noted and decried by Porter Goss [R-FL], the principal congressional sponsor of Ricky Ray, whose initial version of the bill went nowhere [Siplon 2002:62]). Adding insult to injury, final passage of Ricky Ray on October 21, 1998 (the last day of that session of Congress) was entirely drowned out by the rapidly developing Monica Lewinsky scandal. There was no media circus surrounding the passage of Ricky Ray, nor was there serious political pressure either for or against it.

Ricky Ray was a boy with hemophilia who—like Ryan White in Indiana— became infected with HIV and (along with his two brothers) was expelled from school. When—in August 1987—the family obtained a court order ordering the boys' readmission, their home was burned to the ground, and the case became—temporarily—a national sensation. The Ray family were constituents of Porter Goss, a conservative Republican congressman from Florida. Goss took on the Ray case and, more broadly, the cause of HIV-infected hemophiliacs as almost a personal crusade. He played a key role in instigating the IOM report on HIV and the blood supply and—in concert with (by that time) highly mobilized hemophiliacs (Ricky's mother prominent among them)—in securing the passage of the eponymous Ricky Ray Act. It is no accident, of course, that the two principal pieces of U.S. federal legislation in support of persons with HIV/AIDS were named for "innocent" (and presumed heterosexual) boys.[24] Paradoxically, both (most notably Ricky Ray) were passed in a period of vocal political demand for fiscal constraint and with the ardent (and somewhat lonely) support of arch-conservative lawmakers.

Ryan White and Ricky Ray provided political cover for conservative lawmakers in the United States to support funding for persons with HIV/

---

[24] This was strikingly exemplified during an appearance of several boys with hemophilia and AIDS on the Phil Donohue TV show on October 1, 1993. Donohue went out of the way to emphasize that these boys did not have "boyfriends." They were "normal," "heterosexual" males, who played sports and went to school (Davidson 2008:51–52).

AIDS. In the mid-1980s, however, fear of AIDS was at its height, and these boys had yet to become poster children in the AIDS wars. The impact on families with a hemophiliac son, brother, or father of seeing—even at a distance—the stigma, harassment, and worse directed at anyone known or even believed to have AIDS was devastating. A Roper poll conducted in 1985 showed that fully 94% of respondents would either "fight to have the AIDS child removed from school" or "keep your own child home" if they learned that a child with AIDS was attending the same school. The mother of a six-year-old boy with hemophilia recounted her refusal to have him tested for HIV, telling her pediatrician: "Don't make him a potential victim of fear and discrimination" (DePrince 1995:80). Fear that disclosure not only of AIDS but also of hemophilia itself would expose them to discrimination and stigma is clearly reflected in the retrospective comments of men interviewed for Resnik's study of the National Hemophilia Foundation (NHF):

"If any memory prevails [from that period], it is the memory of fear of discrimination."

"[When I became active in the NHF] I did not report that my wife died of AIDS or that I had AIDS because I was a minister and it would be devastating particularly in the South, looking at this as being so leprous and so contagious."

"Nobody with hemophilia wanted anyone to think they might have gotten the disease because they had a gay relationship. . . . I guess people with hemophilia recognized the prejudice that was given to people who were gay with AIDS and didn't want any part of that."[25]

"As an 'epidemiologically significant' group, hemophiliacs were interpellated into homophobic racist discourses for which they were ill prepared" (Davidson 2008:40).

The immediate consequence of this "interpellation" was a policy and practice of nondisclosure. We have described earlier NHF members' response to a proposed "white paper" speaking frankly about AIDS and hemophilia, but it is worth repeating. The paper was "resoundingly" voted down: "The chapters [of AFH], when they saw this white paper, just got up in arms and said, you

---

[25] Comments are drawn from oral history interviews conducted by Susan Resnik and deposited in the Hemophilia Oral History Collection 1987–1998, Columbia Center for Oral History. For further information and context see Resnik (1999).

can't do this, we have people living in this community, if they're exposed their house could be destroyed, this will happen, that will happen, they'll be kicked out of school" (oral history, Resnik Archives, May 1, 1997). Fear of disclosure was accompanied—paradoxically—by active resistance to the quest for compensation. In a 1988 memo, the executive director of NHF wrote: "It is highly unlikely that compensation could ever be considered for all individuals exposed to HIV—this has not occurred in any of the other countries that have initiated or are considering compensation programs. Thus any compensation strategy . . . would be an ideological throw-back to Elizabethan Poor Laws, with notions of deserv[ing] and undeserv[ing] populations. . . . Further this notion of deserv[ing] innocent victims would . . . trigger a major outcry and declaration of war from the gay community" (cited in Bayer 1999:46). This latter comment reflects the domination at that time of AIDS politics in the United States by organized gay men, demanding that not only identities but also politics and policies be constructed with the potential power of gay bodies in mind.

Ryan White and Ricky Ray were categorized first as innocent children and only secondarily as hemophiliacs. Beyond its (presumably self-evident) "innocence," how they came to be infected with AIDS was not seriously addressed in the human-interest stories around these young boys. Far from galvanizing a protest movement, their widely reported horror stories had the opposite effect of demobilizing American hemophiliacs, forcing them back into their medical closets at the very point in time when Garvanoff was taking the first steps toward organized protest by hemophiliacs in France. Collective action would come in the United States but with a lag of several years accounted for by obstacles in political culture and organization unique to the United States.

A dominant theme of AIDS/hemophilia narratives during the late 1980s was the construction of boundaries: between gays and straights, between people with and without AIDS, between hemophiliacs and gays, between innocent/deserving and not-so-innocent/undeserving victims. These boundaries were drawn, and contested, very differently in France than in the United States. The French public's first knowledge of AIDS was as a mysterious disease come from afar that afflicted gay men in the United States (Herzlich and Pierret 1988). And most of the first few French cases were—as in the United States—among gay men.[26] Vocabulary identifying AIDS with

---

[26] Not exclusively, however. Among the early French cases were heterosexual men who had traveled in sub-Saharan Africa and at least one woman (Leibowitch 1984).

gays crossed the Atlantic—"*cancer gay*," "*syndrome gay*"—and there was no lack of moral "othering" of persons with AIDS, documented in Herzlich and Pierret's analysis of French newspaper coverage of the epidemic during the early to mid-1980s. Nevertheless, counternarratives were quick to surface. The very same newspapers that wrote of gay cancer called attention to "Anglo-Saxon Puritanism" and "Reaganism" as responsible for Americans' putative fixation on AIDS as the "just punishment" for homosexuality. The earliest advocates for attention to the epidemic in France were not associations of gay men—who had no traction in the AIDS public space at that time—but a small group of clinicians and medical researchers. These physicians—several of whom were gay themselves—were recognized in the media and, eventually, by French health authorities as legitimate sources of scientific expertise. Their public commitment to refusal of stigmatization or moral judgment of persons whom they identified simply as "patients" was exemplified by their denunciation of "othering" (*mis à l'écart*) in any form (with specific reference to the treatment of Ryan White in the United States). In a similar vein, the founding principle of AIDES, France's largest association organized to provide health and social support to persons with HIV/AIDS was inclusion—that is, although it was started (in 1984) by gay men, it was very deliberate in neither identifying as a gay organization nor in distinguishing among the persons it served according to their sexual and/or gender identity (see, e.g., Pinnell 2002). By 1988, "inclusion" had become the official stated policy of the French government in the AIDS domain.

The early actions of AIDES and of the small "outsider" group of AIDS doctors happened for the most part under the government's radar. It was the intervention of the extreme right political party of Jean-Marie Le Pen—the Front National—in 1986 that pushed AIDS onto the political stage in France and forced the government and mainstream politicians of both left and right to take a stand on the draconian—and highly discriminatory—measures to segregate AIDS patients proposed by Le Pen (Mathiot 1992, Péchu 1992). With almost no political opposition, government officials moved to deliberately and publicly erase the boundaries that the Front National had attempted to construct: there would be no stigmatization of *groupes à risque*, no obligatory screening (with the exception of blood donations), and no separate hospital facilities for AIDS patients. Claude Evin who took over as minister of health in 1988 made the government's position crystal clear: "A deadly epidemic like AIDS carries in itself the germ of exclusion. The fears created by spread of this disease risk triggering rejection of sero-positives and of the sick. Demagogues will play on these fears to try and impose their version of the social and moral order. More than ever, we must reaffirm the solidarity and dignity of our society" (Evin 1988).[27] There were no lack of sob stories about children with AIDS and their grieving parents in the French press and on television. And there was stigma attached to gay men and to persons with AIDS in France as in the United States. But public hostility had been delegitimized and its political base marginalized—at least temporarily. The daunting obstacles to mobilization experienced by hemophiliacs in the United States were largely absent in France.

Mobilization was triggered in the United States when in the early 1990s men with hemophilia and AIDS started talking to each other outside the framework of NHF.[28] Among the many things that angered these men was the NHF's stubborn opposition to the quest for compensation: "The fact that the Compensation Committee that the [AHF] Foundation Board had put together had come back with a recommendation that we not go after compensation—that it was impossible to achieve—pissed us off to no end" (oral history 1997, Resnik Archives). Once the inside revolution in the leadership of NHF had been accomplished in 1994 (see Chapter 5), compensation for hemophiliacs in some form, whether through the courts or the government, became one of the association's principal goals. As we stated at the beginning of this chapter, whether and how a government offers compensation for injuries that occur within its territory are the outcome of competing causal stories—competing portrayals of "facts" and of the moral implications of those facts. The stories told by witnesses in the course of two congressional hearings on the Ricky Ray Act exemplify such stories, in particular the ideological and political resources available to policy actors in the United States that both contributed to and constrained their narrative possibilities.

Witnesses in support of the Ricky Ray Act fell into three categories: "victims"—persons with AIDS or their grieving relatives; associations of hemophiliacs; and the two members of Congress—Goss and De Wine—responsible for introducing the bill in the House and Senate, respectively. Other witnesses included more or less neutral (or performing as neutral) legal and medical "experts" and members of the current (Clinton) administration and, finally, a more hostile group of blood bankers and

[27] French citizenship as an overriding identity and basis for solidarity with other citizens was a founding post-revolutionary principle of the French state (Duchesne 1984).

[28] This is, of course, a more or less exact replication of what had happened in France ten years earlier.

pharmaceutical representatives. The audience for these performances were a very small and shifting number of subcommittee members, the witnesses themselves (when they were not speaking), and a large and occasionally vocal crowd of hemophiliacs and their allies. The latter came from all over the country not just to attend the hearing but also to rally outside the Capitol and lobby their individual members of Congress. Unfortunately, there was no *New Yorker* or *Le Monde* reporter present to fully convey the atmosphere of these occasions. However, according to a description by the *Philadelphia Inquirer* of the bill's final passage in the House: "With the House gallery full of supporters, the voice vote came after about a dozen representatives spoke passionately in favor of passage" (Shaw 1998).

Supporters' narratives followed a consistent pattern. They invariably opened with wrenching stories of agonizing death and devastated families and moved inexorably to the causal connection with government malfeasance: "families whose lives have been torn apart because our Government failed us."[29] Key to these narratives was the moral status of "victims" (as they were described) and of their claims: "innocent" victims, "needlessly" infected, "through no fault of their own," to whom the government had a "moral obligation." In this telling, the government "caused" the problem— hemophiliacs' HIV/AIDS—and was therefore responsible for "fixing" it. The IOM report—*HIV and the Blood Supply*—published in 1995 shortly before the first Ricky Ray hearing was the principal resource for these narratives, and, indeed, it seems unlikely based on these hearings that the Ricky Ray bill would have been proposed or advanced in Congress without that report. Much like the Lucas report in France, it served as authoritative "scientific" grounds for supporters' claims of moral obligation. For example:

An independent scientific review panel (the Institute of Medicine at the National Academy of Sciences) concluded that the government missed opportunities to protect the public health during that period. The IOM found a "failure of leadership and inadequate institutional decisionmaking processes," concluding that the government agencies "consistently chose the least aggressive option that was justifiable." (U.S. House of Representatives 1996:23 [Testimony of Congressman Porter Goss]).

---

[29] U.S. House of Representatives 1996:1.

The last phrase, that government agencies "consistently chose the least aggressive option that was justifiable," was cited not only by congressional supporters but also by witnesses from the hemophilia community. Opponents of Ricky Ray—or at least of its rationale—cited the report as well and were equally selective, calling attention to its more cautionary statements, for example: "The danger of hindsight is unfairly finding fault with decisions that were made in the context of great uncertainty" (Reilly 1995:182).[30] Secretary Shalala had in fact used the latter quotation in earlier congressional testimony following publication of the IOM report, signaling the evident reluctance of the Clinton administration to wholeheartedly endorse Ricky Ray.

The NHF memo cited earlier, warning against the construction of boundaries between deserving and undeserving populations, was nothing if not prescient. Construction of moral boundaries around hemophiliacs that would exclude other potential claimants for government compensation was from the perspective of its supporters in Congress a political sine qua non. "An aide to Representative Porter Goss . . . a conservative Republican committed to budgetary restraint, simply noted, 'If you increase the numbers [i.e., by adding arguably the next most deserving category, persons with transfusion-acquired AIDS] you increase the cost'" (Bayer 1999:48). Senator De Wine made essentially the same argument: "It was our view that the bill would have been defeated if it got complicated by the whole transfusion question, and the hemophiliac group needed and deserved help right away" (Kaufman 2001:3). The hearing record made clear that Goss's and De Wine's congressional colleagues were intensely concerned about setting a "precedent" for others to demand compensation. So hemophiliacs painted themselves and were portrayed as unique: suffering *families* untainted by the sin of "risky" behavior, and patriotic Americans precluded by blood shield laws from seeking justice in the courts. "Within a national AIDS narrative," as Davidson points out, "hemophiliacs played (unwittingly in some cases) an important role in securing an image around which legislation, research, and public policy could be made without having to engage issues of homosexuality and homophobia" (1998:51).[31] The chair of the cognizant committee

---

[30] Manufacturers' representatives went substantially beyond cautionary statements to dispute the factual basis of the IOM report (something that representatives of the U.S. government did not do). It is important to point out that there was no legitimate public venue in France for manufacturers to state their case. First, they were identified with the "government," second, they had been totally discredited well before the issues were even publicly joined.

[31] They played exactly the same role—with even less relation to reality—in passage of the earlier Ryan White Act.

in the Senate, James Jeffords (R-VT) was vocally and actively disturbed by what he believed a totally unwarranted distinction between hemophilia- and transfusion-acquired AIDS, but he was ultimately persuaded: hemophiliacs had a strong grassroots movement and powerful friends in Congress; persons with transfusion-acquired AIDS had neither.

A principal concern voiced by leaders of the NHF had been that a campaign to compensate hemophiliacs would "trigger a major outcry and declaration of war from the gay community" (op. cit.). In truth, the larger AIDS epidemic went virtually unnoticed in the Ricky Ray hearings and in its (scant) coverage by the press; gays were present only by implication as the unmentionable other. Although the AIDS Action Council—the principal Washington lobbying group for gay organizations—did not endorse Ricky Ray (despite the fact that NHF was a member), *POZ Magazine*, a widely read popular magazine on AIDS politics, devoted its January 1, 1997, issue to highly sympathetic articles on the Ricky Ray Act and hemophilia more broadly, treating hemophiliacs as simply one part of the larger community of persons with AIDS. Nevertheless, this sympathy was not universal:

[The Ricky Ray Act] has strong conservative support because it presents politicians with a fantastic opportunity to say that they've done something about AIDS without actually having to help the already-marginalized populations at greatest risk: women, IV-drug users, people of color, the homeless, and gay and bisexual men. Implicit in COTT's demand for federal compensation is the repellent notion that there are innocent AIDS victims (hemophiliacs) and those who brought it on themselves (the rest of us). (Letter to the editor, *POZ Magazine*, March 1, 2000)

There had, indeed, been acknowledged homophobia among hemophiliacs and—as we documented earlier—active efforts both private and public to erect boundaries against identification with gays. Sites of potential identity for persons with AIDS—specifically gay and not gay—long preceded hemophiliacs' grassroots organization and could not go unrecognized, both because of their power in popular culture at the time and—equally important—because of the preexisting political power of gay organizations in the United States. *POZ*'s 1997 issue reflected militant hemophiliacs' recognition of those political realities and their—at least somewhat successful—effort to convert gay men from enemies at worst and suspicious onlookers at best into allies in a common cause.

The Politics of Inclusion and Exclusion

"Victims" (a highly contested label) of HIV/blood contamination were compensated much earlier, more generously, and more inclusively in France than in the United States. Nevertheless, the two countries had a surprising number of points in common. Grassroots movements of hemophiliacs were central to the outcome in both cases, their key role fully acknowledged by the legislations' political sponsors. Second, those sponsors were equally concerned about the legislative "precedent" that compensation might set and—consequently—were equally insistent on the "exceptional" character of the legislative project in question. Finally, despite considerable rhetoric in both countries' legislative bodies pointing the finger at the state and its agencies as "responsible" for the HIV/blood disaster among recipients of contaminated blood, in neither case did this rhetoric make it into the final bill.[32]

These similarities are deceptive, however. The meanings each country's legislators infused into words like "precedent," "exceptional," and "responsibility," the stories they wove around those words, and the conclusions they drew were not the same. As Swidler observed, "culture influences action . . . by shaping a repertoire or 'tool kit' of habits, skills, and styles from which people construct 'strategies of action' " (1986:273). French and American legislators worked with very different political "toolkits." Those toolkits not only shaped their strategies of action but also constrained them.

Claude Got, among the most prominent spokespersons for public health in France, had very little to say about hemophiliacs in his influential 1988 report on the AIDS epidemic prepared at the request of Claude Evin. What Got did say was telling:

> The problem of legal responsibility presented by [transfusion AIDS cases] is difficult to resolve. In analogous situations (contamination by the hepatitis virus, nosocomial infections . . .) compensation has never been

---

[32] This absence had no impact on public interpretation of these legislative acts. They were read by the media and by later commentators in both countries as acknowledgment of government responsibility.

considered. . . . Whatever the solution, *it cannot be limited to HIV* but extended to all problems of the same type, whether that would involve amplifying the notion of legal responsibility or instituting a "solidarity fund" for these situations." (Got 1988:82–83, emphasis added)

Got made the same point in testimony to the Senate Commission of Inquiry into the French transfusion system: "The principle of compensation limited to transfusion-acquired AIDS to the exclusion of other contamination risks was," in his view, "inadmissible" (Sourdille and Huriet 1992:176). Got's perspective is of a piece with prominent officials' denigration of "exclusion" and affirmation of "solidarity" with all AIDS victims.[33] It is a perspective with which both ministerial and parliamentary advocates on behalf of compensation for persons with HIV/AIDS from contaminated blood were forced to contend and with which they had considerable difficulty.

Every participant in French parliamentary debate on the compensation law wrestled with Got's question of how HIV was—morally—different from hepatitis, also acquired from contaminated blood and blood products, or from hospital-acquired iatrogenic infections or, for that matter, from other forms of medical malpractice ("therapeutic accidents"). Their underlying concerns were threefold. First, these concerns reflected a widely shared belief that there was no moral difference—that the correct analogy to HIV contamination was, in fact, with common *"accidents thérapeutiques"* and not with "exceptional" disasters. Second, debate participants were haunted by the fear that in enacting the compensation law they would create a legal "precedent" for holding physicians and hospitals strictly liable (i.e., liable without fault) for harms to patients, leading to a vast expansion in malpractice suits (an outcome uniformly labeled a *"dérive à l'américaine"*) thereby both annoying politically powerful doctors and threatening (asserted the parliamentary *rapporteur* on this legislation) to bankrupt the healthcare system. Third, Parliament was at the end of its current session, it was just before Christmas, and the government was under intense political pressure to come up with a solution quickly. Ending the debate, Minister of Health Bianco wrapped it up as follows:

We must take care that this exceptional risk that resulted in exceptional harm, does not result in legislation that could be applied in circumstances

[33] And it is consistent with the broader French ideology emphasizing citizens' equality of membership in a "universal" national community to the relative exclusion of more particularistic identities (see, e.g., Duchesne 1997).

other than those the legislature intended. The foundation of this compensation is the exceptional character of the risk. (Sénat 1991b&c:5394)

Bianco went on to say, however, reflecting his and his colleagues' political sensitivity to the principle of inclusion that, indeed, "it will be necessary in the future to come up with a project that addresses the entire body of therapeutic risks and accidents" (Sénat 1991b&c:5394). This initiative was adopted as a priority by Bianco's immediate successor, Bernard Kouchner; the requisite legislation was passed in 2002 during Kouchner's second term as minister of health.[34]

American legislators had no comparable qualms about excluding (what they defined as) competing claimants from the reach of Ricky Ray. Hemophiliacs were portrayed and portrayed themselves in congressional hearings as *singularly* afflicted and therefore singularly entitled—a form of political theater that had no counterpart in France. Hemophiliacs with AIDS and/or their family members did not appear as witnesses in any of the French parliamentary forums that addressed the AIDS/blood crisis. Efforts by a single American senator to include individuals with transfusion-acquired AIDS in the Ricky Ray bill were quashed as a political poison pill.[35] Finally, in a partial echo of French concerns with therapeutic accidents, the IOM report had recommended "establishing a no-fault compensation system for individuals who suffer adverse consequences from the use of blood or blood products" (IOM 1995:224). This recommendation had been raised by representatives of the hemophiliac community with their congressional advocates and was alluded to in congressional hearings but received no support and had no afterlife. Exclusion—limiting compensation to hemophiliacs—was justified by personal human-interest stories familiar to American media consumers and carried no political costs.

---

[34] Although Kouchner did not manage to pass this legislation in his first term as minister of health, his seriousness in confronting the problem of what in the United States we would call medical malpractice—and the overall seriousness with which this issue was addressed following the HIV/blood affair in France—is indicated by the influential report he commissioned as minister in 1992–1993: *Le problème Français des accidents thérapeutiques: enjeux et solutions* by François Ewald (Paris: Ministère de la Santé et de l'action humanitaire, 1993). Kouchner's ultimate success is an instance of the profound influence of the HIV/blood affair (and of the AIDS epidemic more generally) in reimagining and expanding the political and policy domain of public health in France.
[35] The reasons alleged for this failure were not only monetary—"If you increase the numbers you increase the cost"—but also the supposed difficulty of proving that claims from transfusees were not a cover for "risky" behavior. It probably did not help that the IOM report was devoted exclusively to the impact of HIV/blood contamination on hemophiliacs and had nothing to say about persons infected by blood transfusion.

8

Authoritative Retrospection

"Authoritative" narratives of the blood affair were produced in France by IGAS (Inspection Générale des Affaires Sociales), better known as the Lucas report; by the French Senate and (separately) by the French Assemblée Nationale (AN); and in the United States by the Institute of Medicine (IOM). These narratives have in common their focus on events in the period 1981–1985 before measures to protect the blood supply—routine HIV testing of donated blood and heat treatment of blood products intended for hemophiliacs—were instituted in both countries. Both the Lucas and IOM reports focus exclusively on the experience of hemophiliacs, ignoring transfusion-associated AIDS. Not only are there parallels in empirical findings among these four reports, but their diagnoses of catastrophe bear a striking resemblance to those of earlier official commission reports on other catastrophes: crises were foreseeable and could have been mitigated; obstacles to effective intervention were rooted in existing structures and cultural traditions; and decisions and actions of elite leaders contributed to negative outcomes (Vaughan 2006).

In almost every other respect the French and American reports were quite different: in the circumstances they were produced, in their authors, and in how these authors understood—or appeared to understand—the task in front of them. The French reports were initiated, carried out, and published in mid-crisis (1991–1993) born of the immediate political imperative to address an unfolding drama that was shaking the nation to its core. No immediate crisis or imperative drove the IOM report published in 1995 two years after hemophiliacs had requested a congressional investigation into HIV contamination of the blood supply and over ten years after the events documented in the report. The first two French reports (Lucas and the Senate) were more or less dramatic accounts of malfeasance; the third, and last (AN) report, a (largely failed) attempt to dedramatize and reinterpret the "facts" alliterated by the earlier reports. The American report reads, in contrast, as a relatively cold-blooded academic analysis of unfortunate policy choices. On a scale of moral outrage ranging from minimum to maximum,

The Social Production of Crisis. Constance A. Nathanson and Henri Bergeron, Oxford University Press.
© Oxford University Press 2023. DOI: 10.1093/oso/9780197682487.003.0008

the IOM and AN reports are at the first extreme, the French Senate report at the second, and the Lucas report somewhere in-between these two
extremems.[1] Underlying the contrasting reports are differences in interests
and incentives of their authors, in policy opportunities afforded by amplification versus mitigation of drama, and in available cultural repertoires.

France

The first of these reports in time, authored by Michel Lucas and known as the
Lucas report, was published on September 10, 1991. Lucas was the inspector
general of IGAS, an arm of the French state with broad government oversight
responsibility in its domain of health and social security either on request by
ministers or on its own initiative. IGAS is an important administrative entity,
staffed by future cabinet members and other government officials, and its
words are taken seriously. The day after its appearance, the Lucas report was
described by Le Monde as the first report on the blood affair "under official
seal" (Nouchi and Nau 1991b). It was also the most influential of the French
reports, treated by judges in the many trials to come as the definitive account
of the blood affair (Beaud 1999:661).

The report had been requested on June 10, 1991, by Jean-Louis Bianco,
minister of social affairs, and Bruno Durieux, minister of health under
Bianco (ministre délégué). The language of their request was significant: "We
want information allowing the precise and exhaustive establishment of the
reality and chronology of facts and decisions taken in this period [1985]
in the blood transfusion domain insofar as they concern hemophiliacs"
(Lucas 1991: Exhibit 1). Their comments to journalists at the time suggest
that these ministers believed a "factual" report would calm turbulent waters stirred up by the French press.[2] The same message was conveyed by
the first sentences of Lucas's introduction to his report: "Time and again
in 1987, 1989, and in the last few months, the press has with increasing intensity raised questions about the conditions under which the security of
transfusion was assured during the first years of AIDS, and more precisely

---

[1] Saul presents a rather different analysis of these reports, stating: "Although the French Senate report and the IOM report were issued three years apart, they looked remarkably similar" (2004:123).
We strongly disagree.

[2] See, e.g., "Jean-Louis Bianco s'explique," Figaro, June 11, 1991; "Un entretien avec M. Bruno
Durieux," Le Monde, June 7, 1991.

between 1983 and 1985" (Lucas 1991:1). The introduction continues with further details of press attacks leading to the resignation of Garretta as director of the Centre National de Transfusion Sanguine (CNTS) and loss of confidence in "our transfusion system" (Lucas 1991:1). The implication is clear that "presenting only facts supported by written documents" would assuage passions and calm tempers aroused by an out-of-control press. Lucas ended his introduction with the claim that his purpose was not to assign responsibility but to analyze the reasons why "decisions were made, not made, or made late." The two subsequent French reports and the report of the IOM made similar disclaimers with equally little influence on how these reports were interpreted by their diverse and highly interested audiences: the bad guys were easily identifiable, whether as worthy of scorn or unfairly targeted.

The Lucas report consisted of sixty-three pages of text and sixty-nine pages of original documents—internal memos, reports, letters, and other communications—dating from August 25, 1983, through December 31, 1987. Although the ministers' request referred only to 1985, the report has two sections. The first section is titled "1981–1984: A Menace Misunderstood (*méconnue*) Overturns Certainties and Hopes"; the second, "1985: A Strategy Is Gradually Put in Place." Lucas used the annexed documents and other sources (principally the U.S. CDC along with selected citations from scientific journals, e.g., *Lancet, New England Journal of Medicine*) to weave a chronological narrative of the "facts." The narrative was sober and restrained in its language, but its appearance of neutrality was deceptive, prefigured by the title of the first section: "Foreseeable Danger Was Unforeseen, Shattering Hopes and Dreams." The title did not specify *whose* hopes and dreams, leaving the reader to assume the widest possible application. Through the effective use of variations in font size and bolding and the juxtaposition of statements by various authorities, Lucas conveyed not so much that knowledge was uncertain as that it was suppressed or unheard. For example, on May 24, 1983, an American blood products manufacturer wrote to CNTS proposing a heat-treated product approved by the FDA. Lucas observed that "this letter apparently received no response" (Lucas 1991:12). On the next page, he cited a 1983 study by CNTS showing that French (not just American) blood products transmitted AIDS. Lucas wrote, "on the objection that the title of this study [that included the phrase 'relative to AIDS'] might be seen by hemophiliacs, the title was changed to refer only to hepatitis" (Lucas 1991:13). Under the heading, "Medical Wager, Marked by a Reassuring Estimate of the Danger," Lucas used large and bolded font to highlight statements by renowned blood authorities to the 1983 annual meeting of the French association of hemophiliacs downplaying the threat of AIDS and the effectiveness of heat treatment. These rhetorical strategies implied at best ignorance and at worst concealment of a known risk. The culprits Lucas identified are blood bankers and principally Michel Garretta, the (by then) former director of CNTS. Only in the concluding pages of his report did Lucas insist that his evaluation of decisions in the blood affair was grounded in scientific knowledge at the time (i.e., 1981–1985) and not in the light of knowledge in 1991. The day following the report's release, Le Monde commented that its "very restrained conclusions in no way permit the identification of any one uniquely responsible for a drama that has its origin at many levels. Individual mistakes, bureaucratic sluggishness, ambiguous ties between hemophiliacs and their physicians, and dysfunctional relations between blood bankers and politicians are all in question" (Nau and Nouchi 1991b).

Not everyone was equally enthralled with the Lucas report. In his book published in 1999, Le Sang contaminé: Essai critique sur la criminalisation de la responsabilité des gouvernants (Contaminated Blood: Critical Essay on the Criminalization Of Political Responsibility), Olivier Beaud, professor of constitutional law at the Sorbonne, made three points. First, Lucas ignored the actions of government ministers; second, he missed important documents (e.g., cabinet archives); and third, and most important, he made two serious factual errors: first in the date when actionable scientific information was available (contested throughout all French [and American] reports and judicial proceedings); and, second, in "insinuating" that approval of the American Abbott test was delayed for "commercial and economic" reasons. Commercial and economic motives became from then on, asserts Beaud, the lens through which the "prosecutors" (i.e., media and the courts) viewed the entire blood affair (1999:677). Indeed!

If the goal of Bianco and Durieux was to calm troubled waters, they were to be disappointed. Not only did journalistic attention to the blood affair explode following publication of the Lucas report (increasing fourfold in Le Monde alone) but also the tenor of coverage quickly moved to accusing the report itself and the ministers who requested it of "concealment": ministers promised transparency; the report was incomplete; documents were hidden. At the same time, former ministers and officials launched accusations at one another, and the French Senate launched its own investigation.

On October 30, 1991, the Senate proposed a "mission of information" on blood transfusion.[3] The proposal—advanced by four of the Senate's committees—was adopted without objection on November 15. The investigation played out over five months with some forty witnesses, modeled explicitly on a U.S. congressional hearing. Its aims were "to study the technical, administrative, and financial management of blood transfusion in France and the means for its improvement, notably with respect to the principals of voluntary (*don bénévole*) blood donation" (Sénat 1991a:3775). In 1991 (and through March 1993), the government in power was Socialist, but the Senate was in the hands of conservatives, and over half the commission's members belonged to one or another of several conservative parties.[4] The commission was led by two highly prominent conservative Senators (Jacques Sourdille and Claude Huriet). Eight of the commissions twenty-one members were physicians by profession, including both Sourdille and Huriet.[5]

Condemnation of the French blood system introduced Lucas's report but was placed in the words of journalists. The Senate report's introduction condemned the system first hand in scathing terms signed by the commission's president: "Absence of transparency in the blood system, blind assertions by celebrated and/or powerful physicians, ambitions for an industrial empire, typically nationalist pretensions of research institutions, incorrect and quasi-ideological references to the rights of man justifying rejection of screening tests and donor selection would combine to perpetuate the distribution of contaminated blood to trusting recipients" (Sourdille and Huriet 1992:7).[6] There followed a detailed account of what was described

---

[3] It should be kept in mind that under the Constitution of the Fifth Republic, the French Senate (and the French Parliament overall) has substantially less power in relation to the executive branch than their counterparts in the United States (see, e.g., Cerny and Schain 1980, Andrews and Hoffmann 1981). Claude Huriet had substantial prestige as an individual.

[4] The precise role of party affiliation in shaping the Senate's approach to its investigation is murky. As Pinell pointed out, moral outrage aroused by the blood affair transcended political parties (2002:250). Further, the dominance of physicians in the Senate restrained its members from going too far in their attacks on blood bankers, hematologists, and treaters of hemophiliacs, all of whom were physicians. At the same time, French politics in this period were extremely unsettled. Mitterrand, a Socialist, had been president of France since 1981 and would continue in that role until 1995. But over the period 1985–1995, the National Assembly and, hence, the government switched between Socialist and conservatives twice (including in the spring of 1993). The Senate was in conservative hands throughout.

[5] Physicians have long had a prominent place in French political life (see Nathanson 2007).

[6] The Senate report was published in the *Journal Officiel de la République* (*JOR*, similar to the Congressional Record) on June 12, 1992. It was published as a book under the authorship of Sourdille and Huriet shortly thereafter. Our quotes and page references are from the book version and cited accordingly. "Incorrect and quasi-ideological references to the rights of man" was a barely veiled reference to gay groups' objection to screening blood donors.

throughout the report as "the drama" of contaminated blood, its origins in individual and institutional failures, along with proposals for reform. Consistent with Mary Douglas's observation on cultural debates about risk and justice that "anyone who insists that there is a high degree of uncertainty is taken to be opting out of accountability" (Douglas 1992:30), the Senate commission made clear on the first page of its report what it thought about claims of scientific uncertainty: "If spring 1985 marked the fixed date of certainty and of unmitigated (*inexpiables*) responsibilities, multiple cries of alarm were sounded two years earlier" citing Montagnier, Gallo, and other scientific authorities (Sourdille and Huriet 1992:7). Testimony by witnesses (e.g., the president of France's equivalent of the AMA) that ideas about AIDS in 1985 were "incomplete or mistaken" were ignored. In the commission's reading, the science was there—not so much deliberately concealed (as in Lucas), but unseen.[7]

The Senate commission's indictment of the French blood system had two threads: first, its "sacralization" and its prestige ("the best in the world") blinded blood bankers and government officials not only to the emerging threat of HIV in the blood supply but also to the system's ongoing financial, managerial, and quality control problems;[8] second, as stated in one of the report's chapter headings, "Ambition Informed by Industrial Logic Led to Forgetting the Rules of Medical Ethics" (Sourdille and Huriet, 1992:45). Multiple witnesses argued that CNTS was the victim of its entrepreneurial ambitions. Nevertheless, the near impossibility of reconciling senators' and witnesses' constantly reiterated devotion to the ethical principles of a voluntary and nonprofit blood system with their equally strong desire for an internationally competitive and profitable industry for the manufacture of blood products was evident, for example, in the somewhat astonishing argument that if blood bankers no longer respected ethical imperatives they could at least have acted as good businessmen! "They did neither" asserted the authors of the Senate report (Sourdille and Huriet 1992:48). Ultimately, though, and unsurprisingly, the report held the state at fault, first, for failing to control the blood bankers and, second, for failing to take seriously the

[7] The title of the National Assembly report along with its roster of witnesses suggests a greater attention to scientific uncertainty.

[8] These problems had been identified in IGAS reports from the early 1980s. Their seriousness and CNTS's reluctance to admit and address them is indicated by the fate of the director of CNTS first appointed in 1984 (Jacques Ruffié) to succeed Jacques Soulier (who had been director for thirty years). Ruffié lasted three months, to all appearances as a consequence of calling attention to CNTS's managerial problems.

drama unfolding before its eyes until forced to do so by "parliament, [civil society] associations, and the media." In the undisguised moral outrage of its authors at what they clearly regarded as unconscionable behavior on the part of public officials, the Senate became a principal actor not only in the social production of the French blood crisis but also in the reforms of pharmaceutical regulation, the blood system, and public health more generally that followed over the next decade (Bergeron and Nathanson 2012, Nathanson and Bergeron 2017).

Among the more striking aspects of the third (and last) "official" report on the blood affair in France was its obscurity. This report, from a commission appointed by the AN, titled "Inquiry on the State of Scientific Knowledge and Actions Taken with Respect to the Transmission of AIDS over the Past 10 Years in France and Overseas," was published in the *JOR* on February 5, 1993, almost a year after the Senate report. It was not discussed and barely referenced in the major works on the AIDS/blood crisis in France; it received little or no coverage in France's national newspapers; in the course of searching for a copy of the report, we were told by a scholar of the French blood crisis that it was "politically unimportant." Be that as it may, the AN report in its reliance on eminent scientists as witnesses and its near exclusive emphasis on scientific uncertainties and controversies surrounding the early years of AIDS make it a powerful counterpoint to the Lucas and Senate reports. Much like the anguished plea of French scientists and Nobel laureates to Mitterrand a year later that "expert scientific testimony about the decisions that were made" was not allowed in the Garretta trial, the AN report fell on ears deaf to a narrative that privileged the claims of now delegitimized "scientists."

Formation of the parliamentary commission was itself highly politicized. Faced with intense and well-organized pressure to bring to "justice" (Socialist) government ministers held responsible for the events of 1985, President Mitterrand used a TV address on November 9, 1992, to state that the ministers in question had a right to defend themselves in court (a step leading within the year and under a new, conservative government, to constitutional reform and the creation of a new court competent to try government ministers). From the perspective of the conservative minority in the AN, the proposal to form a commission of inquiry, brought forward by the Socialist majority on November 10, 1993, the day after Mitterrand's address, was a blatant ploy to whitewash these Socialist ministers in advance of any court appearance, and they refused to participate in the commission. (The Senate commission had included members of both parties.) Socialist deputies accused conservatives of being unwilling to face the truth for fear their preconceived opinions would "blow up," and conservatives accused Socialists of hypocrisy.

The AN and Senate commissions took testimony from sixty witnesses altogether, of whom only eight were common to both investigations. These latter included Claude Got (a dominant figure in French public health and author of the first official report on AIDS in France [Got 1989]), Michel Lucas, Jean-Pierre Soulier (immediate predecessor of Garretta as director of CNTS), and Jean-Baptiste Brunet (principal epidemiologist at the DGS during the period 1981–1985). The remaining four individuals interviewed by both commissions were present or former officials of the French transfusion system. The most marked contrast between the AN and the Senate roster of witnesses was the large presence before the AN commission of France's (and the world's) pioneers in the scientific unraveling of AIDS: Luc Montagnier, Willy Rozenbaum, Jean-Claude Chermann, along with other prominent French scientists and physicians (e.g., a Nobel laureate in medicine; the director of INSERM, France's equivalent of the NIH; and others). While we were not able to retrieve the original texts, the AN report contains extended excerpts from their testimony. Once again, none of these individuals were interviewed by the Senate. The AN report also includes excerpts from interviews with prominent authorities in the United States (e.g., Anthony Fauci).

The first section of the AN report is titled, "From Scientific Uncertainty to the Underestimation of Public Health Urgency."[9] The word "uncertainty" (or "uncertainties") is repeated thirteen times in the first nineteen pages of the report. The first twenty pages are devoted to establishing, first, the legitimacy of uncertainty as a scientific posture and, second, the dangers of judging past policy actions based on present scientific knowledge. The "voice" of the AN report is that of its chosen *rapporteur*: summarizing the report's findings in advance, he stated, "the work of the Commission has clearly shown that the question of AIDS in our country as in other industrialized countries has been dominated by many uncertainties that weighed heavily on the disease and on the means of preventing it" (AN 1993:14). This emphasis on uncertainty was reinforced by a series of quotations from the scientific luminaries identified

---

[9] Compare the title of the first section of the Senate report, "The Drama of Blood Contamination in France" (Sourdille and Huriet 1992).

above to the effect that "uncertainty and ignorance are not the same thing," that confirmation of discoveries by multiple scientists is essential ("knowledge that is not shared does not exist"), and that "one must be very modest about certain things that are strongly proclaimed today that were perceived differently at the time." A particularly high-placed mandarin of French science made the point more directly, "I profoundly distrust opinions advanced in 1992 about events that occurred in 1985."

In the body of its report and in the light of this introduction, the AN commission revisited each of the "actions taken" in the "critical period of 1985 for which our country's officials are being taken to task (*mise en cause*)": donor selection, donor testing, and heat treatment of blood products for hemophiliacs. We will use the example of donor selection to illustrate the difference between the tone of the AN report and that of the Senate, published a year earlier. The facts invoked in these two reports are essentially the same: a "circular" dated June 20, 1983, identifying categories of persons "at risk" and calling for donor selection (including exclusion of homosexuals with multiple partners and injection drug users), was prepared by the DGS and addressed to transfusion centers; this circular was essentially a dead letter on arrival: its minimal application was confirmed both by witness interviews and by a survey of transfusion centers, cited by both reports. The treatment of these "facts" was, however, very different. The AN report opened its discussion by calling attention to the rapidity with which this circular was published (just a few weeks after parallel action by the United States and way ahead of other European countries), to the strong support for AIDS surveillance from the Ministry of Health (without which "France would not have discovered the virus in 1983"), and to the "fact" that "this was the only measure possible at the time."

The AN report fully acknowledged that the circular did not have its intended results. This misfortune was explained sympathetically and undramatically: "None of the actors in the transfusion field realized the seriousness of the risk." They saw very few AIDS cases. They were much more concerned about hepatitis than AIDS. They were convinced of the beneficial qualities of "pure" and "unpaid" French blood and transfused it to excess. By clear implication, even if the circular was a dead letter, this was not due to the actions of government ministers but to the inaction of transfusion doctors. The Senate report surrounded much the same explanatory hypotheses with highly dramatic language: "a blindness heavy with consequences" (referring to the underestimation of risk), "a false feeling of security" (referring to

misplaced confidence in French blood), and "the absence of a clear and co-
herent official message" (a point directly contradicted by the AN report's interpretation of actions by the health ministry). In the same vein, controversies
over blood testing and heat treatment held up to scorn by the Senate were
framed by the AN report as reflections of genuine scientific uncertainty and
unexceptional differences of opinion among scientists and physicians in the
face of "continuing lively debate among the most knowledgeable scientists
during the critical period of 1985" (AN:144). Nowhere in the AN report are
the scathing references to deliberate concealment, economic greed, industrial overreach, and organizational failure that are dotted throughout the
earlier report by the Senate.

Given the context of virulent attacks throughout 1991 and 1992, directed
initially at officials of the transfusion system and rapidly extended to the entire (Socialist) political class, it is hard *not* to read the AN report—fairly or
unfairly and despite its heavy scientific authority—as an effort by Socialist
politicians to exonerate their colleagues who had the misfortune to hold
ministerial office during the events of 1985 now (in 1993) broadly interpreted
(by no means only by the Senate) as a betrayal of the French people. Mary
Douglas vividly described the social dynamic at work: "Within the cultural
debate about risk and justice opponents seek to inculpate the other side and
exonerate their own supporters from blame" (1992:30).

United States

In his review of the IOM report in the *American Journal of Public Health*,
Ronald Bayer described its most enduring contribution as the "establishment of a narrative of the events of blood and AIDS in the first years of the
epidemic" (1997:476). The contribution of America's blood system to AIDS
transmission among hemophiliacs and transfusion recipients had been
documented in official reports and the press well before the publication of
the IOM report in 1995 (see Chapter 4). Americans were susceptible to the
heartbreaking stories of *individual* victims, especially if they were portrayed
as asexual children. Neither the detailed reporting of Randy Shilts, nor the
outraged headlines of Gilbert Gaul, nor the sober Dingell hearings had
succeeded in persuading the American public of a crisis in the blood *system*.

At first glance, the contrast between the French reports and *HIV and the
Blood Supply: An Analysis of Crisis Decisionmaking* (the IOM report) were

stark in almost every respect: the IOMs provenance, the composition of the IOM committee charged with the investigation, the political context within which the investigation was launched, and above all, the meaning of the National Academy of Sciences and the IOM as authoritative scientific bodies. Jasanoff observes that "turning to a [scientific advisory] committee for advice" (as was done in this case) "subtly recasts an inherently political judgement about the acceptability of risk as a scientific judgement about the acceptability of evidence" (1990:160), and committees of the National Academy of Sciences are the country's gold standard of scientific advisory bodies. As we noted earlier, there are important parallels between the empirical *findings* of the French and American investigators: conflicts of interest among blood bankers, fragmented policy decision processes, resistance to blood screening among gay men, and others. The difference among these reports is in how these findings were framed, or in what Hilgartner would call the "performance" of these committees (Hilgartner 2000)—Lucas and the (French) Senate of barely restrained anger and outrage, the IOM of disinterested science. The AN "performed" disinterested science as well but for a more or less undisguised political purpose; the IOM was more subtle.

By contrast with the path to the Lucas report, a short one step from health ministers to the inspector general of social affairs, the path to the IOM report was long and convoluted: from newly militant hemophiliacs to members of Congress to the Clinton cabinet member for health (Donna Shalala) to the IOM. Hemophiliacs organized outside of the NHF had begun in 1992 to press for a congressional investigation into the failures that led to the massive infection of American hemophiliacs (Bayer 1999:40). They approached Senator Edward Kennedy and (strategically) Florida Senator Bob Graham and Representative Porter Goss, elected from the district that was home to the Ray family. Much to the anger of militants, their proposal for a congressional investigation was rejected. Although we can only speculate, it is plausible that Democrats feared a full-scale congressional investigation of blood contamination would only provide a larger public platform for Henry Hyde's and Jesse Helms's attacks on gay men as responsible for blood contamination.[10] Instead, Kennedy, Graham, and Goss wrote a joint letter to Shalala dated April 27, 1993, requesting that

---

[10] Dingell's blood supply safety hearings were ongoing at the time but, as we have noted, were focused on the present and future of the blood supply, not its past deficiencies. There is some evidence (to be described below) of a strong desire on the part of Congress (or at least congressional Democrats) to depoliticize the blood affair and to protect the FDA and the CDC. A member of the

the Department of Health and Human Services Office of the Inspector
General investigate the issue of HIV transmission among hemophiliacs
through contaminated   blood products. There are approximately 20,000
hemophiliacs in the United States. Tragically, at least half this population
contracted HIV between 1982 and 1984 from contaminated blood product
transfusions. We ask that you review the events which led to this widespread
transmission of HIV among hemophiliacs, including knowledge within the
public and private sector regarding the possibility of transmission through
blood products and the availability of other non-contaminated products.[11]

Shalala responded with a delay of two months, making it clear that this request would be treated as a "scientific" not a "political" question: "Because a
high level of scientific and medical expertise is required to conduct a thorough study, I have asked that the project be undertaken by the Institute of
Medicine of the National Academy of Sciences." Shalala also repeated a statement made over and over again almost ritually in hearings and reports on the
blood supply: "I am sure you appreciate that the blood supply in the United
States is the safest in the world," and emphasized the utility of this "thorough
study" in "strengthening capacities to ensure the safety of the Nation's blood
supply against new challenges in the *future*" (emphasis added). It is striking
that this correspondence refers exclusively to hemophiliacs as if the "blood
supply" was of concern only to them. At the time of writing in 1993, the CDC
estimated about twice as many cases of transfusion-associated HIV infection
as compared with cases among hemophiliacs.

The fourteen members of the IOM committee were selected for their expertise and for the fact that none had previously spoken on the issues to be
investigated. They included two social scientists; lawyers; an ethicist; and
representatives from the disciplines of biology, medicine, and public health,
all distinguished in their fields. Its aims were straightforward—"to examine the decisions made from 1982 through 1986 to safeguard blood and
blood products, and to evaluate the actions taken to contain the AIDS epidemic"—as were its disclaimers: "This report does not seek to determine

IOM committee characterized Congress as "punting" and the committee's work as "highly sensitive"
and surrounded by "powerful interests."

[11] This letter and its reply are reproduced on pp. 33–34 of the hearing before the House of
Representatives Subcommittee on Human Resources and Intergovernmental Relations, "Protecting
the Nation's Blood Supply from Infectious Agents: New Standards to Meet New Threats," held on
October 12 and November 2, 1995.

liability or affix blame for any individual or collective decisions regarding HIV transmission through blood or blood products during this time period" (IOM 1995:vi). Neither aims or disclaimers were substantially different from statements introducing the three French reports. But the institutional framework—the august reputation of the National Academy of Sciences and the mandate to preserve that reputation—was highly distinctive in its impact on how those aims and disclaimers were interpreted: "The need to stay on mission was reiterated to us by IOM staff and by the committee's chair. . . . It was not the role of the panel to get on one side or another of litigation. . . . What we were doing was framed as 'risk assessment.' It was almost an academic framework. The tragedy at the center (the hemophiliacs) was bounded, put aside" (member of IOM committee, interview by author, March 6, 2019).

The IOM report told a familiar story of delayed and fragmented decision-making, conflicts of interest, and intragovernmental jealousies. Apart from the bureaucratic language and absence of moral outrage, it was in the report's foregrounding of scientific uncertainty and reluctance to attribute responsibility that it departed markedly from the French Senate report and, to a lesser extent, from the Lucas report. On the report's second page—the same location where the Senate report had placed its most vehement denunciations—we read, "The Committee undertook this assignment fully aware of the benefits and risks of hindsight . . . . The risk of hindsight is unfairly finding fault with decisions made by people who had to act long before scientific knowledge became available to dispel their uncertainty" (1995:vi). What in the French reports (excepting the AN report) was ignorance, blindness, or deliberate suppression motivated by greed was described in the American report (and by the AN report) as caution: "There was . . . substantial scientific uncertainty about the costs and benefits of the available options [to reduce the risk of AIDS transmission by blood and blood products]. The result was a pattern of responses which, while *not in conflict with the available scientific information*, were very cautious" (1995:9, emphasis added). "Caution" might, of course, have led to action rather than inaction, particularly in light of the committee's statement on the last page but four of the report that "from early 1983, it was clear that AHF concentrate was a risky product" (1995:231).

It is difficult not to be struck by the convoluted language employed by drafters of the IOM report to avoid direct attributions of responsibility: "The Committee believes it is not possible to conclude that the FDA made a decision that was clearly in the interest of public health given available information as of July 19, 1983" (151); "The Committee has not documented that any actions taken by decisionmakers were inconsistent with their responsibilities" (127). Bayer writing in 1999 described the IOM report as "scathing" in its indictment of (in particular) FDA inaction, and it is clear from the hearing record that the report played a key role in passage of the Ricky Ray Act. Nevertheless, in the choice of venue for investigation of the blood affair, in the charge to the investigating committee, and in its exculpatory language, the IOM report was a powerful act of depoliticization. Despite their role in its initiation and on the opening day of the IOM investigation, the voices of hemophiliacs were almost entirely absent in the report itself. As Kleinman and colleagues observed, "by not addressing what is at stake for the victims—failure to protect patients in an era of increasingly commodified health care—[the IOM report] led to an exculpatory solution that obfuscated the moral dimensions of suffering" (Keshavjeea et al. 2001:1081).[12] Obfuscation carried over into the report's reception by the Department of Health and Human Services (DHHS), the department that had officially requested it, and was reflected in the scant attention its publication received in the American press.[13] Except within a very small circle of stakeholders, publication of the IOM report was a non-event without a significant place on the political or public agenda.

Reflections

Among elements that may have created—or blocked—incentives, resources, and opportunities for authors of these reports to dramatize the blood affair were pre-existing cross-national variations in political context. Critiques of the blood system, of pharmaceutical regulation, and of the overall weakness of public health in France had preceded the HIV/blood affair for years and may have produced incentives—particularly among the conservative parties that dominated the French Senate at the time—for political amplification to

[12] This transformation is all the more striking in light of the public testimony of hemophiliacs that opened the IOM investigation, reducing the panel "to tears and speechlessness by hour after hour of the most tragic and damning testimony" (Keshavjeea et al. 2001:1088) and the intense attention of hemophiliacs to the committee's deliberations, including foregathering outside of the National Academy of Science's headquarters in Washington, D.C.

[13] This lack of notice was documented in our own research and is consistent with comments by other observers (e.g., Starr 2002:338). Michael Stoto (IOM staff member at the time and co-editor of the IOM report) told us that other issues he was working on—Agent Orange and vaccine safety—got much more attention (personal communication, 2019).

precipitate reform. Here was an opportunity to—at the very least—embarrass the Socialist government in power both at the time (in 1991) and also in 1985, when the actions newly identified as scandalous occurred. These same politics doomed the AN report to oblivion. Despite its roster of expert witnesses and the obvious similarities in tone and content to the IOM report, it was born in partisan controversy and had none of the scientific authority commanded by the U.S. National Academy of Sciences and IOM. Further, and probably of more importance, by the time the AN report was published in early 1993, the dominant French narrative of greed and betrayal by government ministers was fully established not only, of course, by the Senate report but also by highly public legal proceedings and media coverage.

When the IOM committee convened in the fall of 1994, Republicans had just taken control of the House of Representatives, and the FDA came under scathing attack (Lewis 1995). The CDC was still reeling from the swine flu affair (Neustadt and Fineberg 1978) and was mired in interagency conflict with the FDA and NIH (IOM 1995). Both agencies had experienced severe budget cuts under the Reagan administration. According to one of its members, the IOM committee was more concerned to protect these agencies than to reform them and had little incentive to amplify perceived failures (IOM committee member, by author, March 6, 2019). Another participant in drafting the IOM report suggested that criticism of 1980s blood policies was a particularly sensitive issue for gays, some of whom had entered the newly elected Clinton administration in 1993 (IOM staff member, interview by author, September 30, 2019). Both the AN and IOM reports dwelt heavily on scientific uncertainty. In France, to invoke uncertainty was interpreted as opting out of accountability, and its advocates were dismissed. In the United States, identical language was interpreted as the sober voice of expert science; it was heavily and selectively quoted in the course of the 1995 congressional hearings on the blood supply by Clinton administration representatives concerned to protect government agencies and by pharmaceutical representatives concerned to deflect blame for their role in blood contamination (U.S. House of Representatives 1995).

A further contrast between the two countries' dominant narratives was in the attribution of responsibility for HIV/blood contamination. Political actors, notes Deborah Stone, "compose stories that describe harms and difficulties, attribute them to actions of other individuals or organizations, and thereby claim the right to invoke government power to stop the harm" (1989:282). Although all four reports invoked government power to do something about the harm caused by contamination of the blood supply, there was a notable difference in their willingness to retrospectively attribute responsibility for causing the harm and/or political responsibility for failing to prevent it: clear and highly concentrated attributions of responsibility in France, vague and widely diffused in the United States. As the sole legitimate policy actor, the state in France not only "owned" the problem of blood contamination in its capacity as the ultimate public health authority but was also held liable for causing the problem and for redressing its consequences.[14] The authors of the IOM report both spread responsibilities far more widely (blood bankers, government agencies, organized hemophiliacs) and invariably mitigated them with language of "scientific uncertainty" and the dangers of retrospective judgment. The example of the AN report demonstrates how little traction this rhetoric had in France.

As the foregoing suggests, there were marked cross-national differences in these reports' framing of scientific uncertainties and interpretation of risks, in the sorts of evidence considered legitimate bases for policy, and in where boundaries were drawn not only between science and politics but also between science and human suffering. Strikingly, differences in framing of scientific uncertainty advanced in the early stages of the epidemic, before the discovery of the virus and institution of effective measures to protect the blood supply, were minimal: blood bankers, regulatory authorities, and organized hemophiliacs in both countries downplayed the risks of blood contamination. Only later, in the throes of the blood crisis, did the French raise questions about the human cost of modern technology and the role of the market in scientific governance, questions that went largely unarticulated and unaddressed in the United States.

---

[14] Gusfield identifies three dimensions of responsibility for public problems: ownership (authority in the relevant field), causal responsibility (how come?), and political responsibility (what is to be done?) (1981:10–14). In France all three dimensions are centered on the state. In the United States, they are spread out and highly contested.

PART III
REFLECTIONS

9

The Social Production of Political Crisis

There are multiple ways to think about our stories of toxic blood. Foremost is the question that animated us from the beginning of this project: Why a crisis in France and not in the United States and what can those different trajectories tell us about the social production of political crises? In this chapter, we draw on our empirical data together with a rich body of recent literature in the social and political sciences to advance a conceptual framework that not only accounts for the divergent pathways taken by France and the United States in response to HIV/blood contamination but also contributes to knowledge of the social processes by which occurrences in the world are transformed into political crises.

In the normal course of events ruptures in the social fabric "are neutralized and reabsorbed into the preexisting structures in one way or another ... forcefully repressed, pointedly ignored, or explained away as exceptions" (Sewell 1996:843). The question of *under what circumstances neutralization fails* and routine turbulence gives way to destabilization and crisis has been central to recent theories of social and institutional change (Seo and Creed 2002, Sewell 1992, 1996, Clemens and Cook 1999, Beckert 2010, Fligstein and McAdam 2012, Alexander 2018, 2019). Each of the conceptual frameworks these scholars propose identifies and elaborates critical *pieces* of this puzzle: the source of destabilization and the setting in which it occurs; individual and/or collective action that pushes the state of play from mere turbulence to "episodes of contention" (Fligstein and McAdam 2012:19); and the transformation of mere "contention" into crisis. To fully understand the social production of political crisis requires that we bring these separate pieces together into a common framework. The framework we propose owes a great deal to the bodies of scholarship cited above but also, and above all, to the detailed case comparison set forth in this book. The reasoning that led us to this framework might be described as theoretically informed induction from the minutiae of empirical data.

Work on institutional change has shifted in recent years from a nearly exclusive emphasis on "exogenous shocks" as transformative disrupters of

The Social Production of Crisis. Constance A. Nathanson and Henri Bergeron, Oxford University Press.
© Oxford University Press 2023. DOI: 10.1093/oso/9780197682487.003.0009 .

institutional fields toward increasing attention to internal contradictions within fields: "ruptures and inconsistencies both among and within the established social arrangements [that generate] tensions and conflicts within and across social systems which may, under some circumstances, shape consciousness and action to change the present order" (Seo and Creed 2002:225). However, as these scholars have noted, inconsistencies and contradictions within or across institutions do not inevitably result in social change: "The question is what triggers particular contradictions to receive attention?" (Thornton et al. 2012:163). To answer this question, we need to specify potential sources of contradiction in the social arrangements that prevail in a given institutional field. These "social arrangements" have been characterized in various ways that almost invariably reduce to some combination of beliefs (cultural schemas, symbolic constructions, cognitive processes) and material practices (social networks, institutional rules).[1] Contradictions within and between beliefs and practices are common. Returning to (and amplifying) the questions raised earlier, under what circumstances do these contradictions (1) rise to the point of visibility in the public sphere and (2) cause unacceptable ruptures that fail to be "neutralized and reabsorbed" into preexisting structures? Equally important, under what circumstances do those same contradictions remain invisible so that no rupture occurs? We propose that the social production of political crisis happens on three levels: first, underlying contradictions in the beliefs and practices that animate an important "field" of action in the polity (see, e.g., Seo and Creed 2002, Clemens and Cook 1999, Beckert 2010, Thornton et al. 2012); second, a process of "strategic mobilization" that renders those contradictions visible in the public arena (see, e.g., Morris 1993, Fligstein and McAdam 2012, Alexander 2018, 2019); and third, a cultural array of beliefs (schemas, symbolic constructions) that frames those contradictions as immoral and unacceptable (Sewell 1992, Benford and Snow 2000). We begin our theoretical argument with a brief recapitulation of the state of play in France and the United States before 1991 when the crisis erupted in France.

---

[1] We acknowledge that this is an oversimplification, particularly in the elements of "material practice." Its purpose is to avoid jargon that may be unfamiliar to our readers. Following the scheme proposed by Jens Beckert, field components include "cognitive frames" (beliefs), "institutions," and "social networks" (material practices) (2010:605). Beckert uses "institutions" to refer to the institutional *rules* that shape a given field and "social networks" to mean the social *relationships* that prevail within the field.

The Field Before the Crisis

In the years before 1991 not only were the identity, resources, and relationships of actors within the field of blood collection and transfusion and between those actors and the state *broadly* similar in France and the United States, but contradictions within the field were comparable as well.[2] France's blood system was nominally (and in French popular understanding) "state run." In fact, the French system was—like that of the United States although on a much smaller scale—privately run, highly fragmented, and internally competitive. As we have described, France ended the Second World War with a chaotic mix of centers engaged in the collection, processing, and transfusion of blood, organized under different administrative auspices and with different organizational forms. There was little or no central coordination or funding and—as in the American case—local blood services were dominated by local medical and lay elites. In both cases, technical oversight was largely in the hands of blood bankers with a strong interest in perpetuating the organizational configurations and services they oversaw. Administrative reports highly critical of what they described as dysfunctional, poorly managed, and inefficient blood "systems" were published in both countries at almost exactly the same time, in the early 1970s, leading to minimal and largely meaningless reforms (Blin et Bestaux 1971, National Research Council 1970). A striking instance of the parallel "logics" of French and American actors in the blood field was their normalization of the risks to hemophiliacs of hepatitis transmitted through blood products: "In the context of the dramatic improvements in the care and treatment of hemophiliacs offered by AHF concentrates, infection associated with the use of these blood products came to be deemed an 'acceptable risk' " (IOM 1995:172); for physicians treating hemophiliacs hepatitis was "an accepted risk, almost all hemophiliacs were contaminated" (Chauveau 2011:122).[3]

Both countries had tightly knit communities of hemophiliacs and established organizations to represent them, and in both cases these organizations

---

[2] Following Fligstein and McAdam, we conceptualize a "field" as a constructed social order "in which actors (who can be individual or collective) are attuned to and interact with one another on the basis of shared (which is not to say consensual) understandings about the purposes of the field, relationships to others in the field (including who has power and why), and the rules governing legitimate action in the field" (2012:9).

[3] Like the Pap-smear, O-rings, and Oxycontin, blood concentrates were deemed the "right tool for the job" (Casper and Clarke 1998); their attendant risks were accepted and "normalized" (Vaughan 1996, Pryma 2022).

maintained close ties not only with their treating physicians but also (in France) with blood donors and (in both countries) with the blood bankers and fractionators that enabled these patients and their families to lead normal lives. In France, the Association Française des Hémophiles (AFH) shared premises with the Centre National de Transfusion Sanguine (CNTS). In the United States, in the late 1970s when the National Hemophilia Foundation (NHF) was going in and out of bankruptcy, it accepted money from blood product manufacturers to fund its activities and welcomed the latter's participation "in summer camps, in workshops that the families attend" and in other ways that went well beyond the mere purveying of a product (Resnik 1999:98). Until 1991 in France, there was no organization in either country to represent the interests of whole blood transfusion recipients.

From CDC's first note on "*Pneumocystis* pneumonia in homosexual men—Los Angeles" published in *MMWR* on June 5, 1981, French infectious disease specialists and virologists were privy to the same scientific information as their American counterparts. Not only scientific and clinical information but also such items as blood policy guidelines from the FDA and the U.S. Department of Health and Human Services were actively shared. Both countries had the same knowledge. And in many respects, responses to that knowledge were the same as well. Both in France and the United States, the first lines of response from blood industry and medical elites were to discount the message, discredit the messenger, and reassure the consumers.[4] And there is little doubt that French no less than American hemophiliacs—whose lives had been "miraculously" saved and rendered livable by blood-clotting factor—were initially disinclined to question that reassurance (see, e.g., IOM 1995, Resnik 1999, Fillion 2009).

Finally, the same or highly similar actions (or inactions) on the part of health authorities that produced scandal and political crisis in France also occurred in the United States, specifically failure to recall toxic or potentially toxic (unscreened or untested) blood and blood products from the market. The 1995 IOM report identified (and analyzed in some detail) two such (in)actions by the FDA: first, the failure to recall blood or blood products that were not collected or produced according to the recommendations it published in early 1983; second, the delay until 1989 to require the recall

---

[4] A well-established pattern in the early response to epidemic fears as described by Charles Rosenberg (1989).

and destruction of non-heat-treated blood when by 1985 heat treatment was accepted as effective in killing the human immunodeficiency virus (HIV). Investigation by the Dingell committee uncovered multiple instances of toxic blood release by Red Cross blood centers extending well into the 1990s.[5]

Translated into the terms of our theoretical framework, French and American blood bankers and manufacturers of blood products in the period before 1991 were embedded in parallel (and indeed partially overlapping) close organizational and personal networks of internal and external exchange—of ideas (scientific, clinical, organizational); practices (medical, public health); and material and symbolic goods (whole blood and blood products). Actors in these networks—blood bankers, regulatory bodies, donors, consumers (i.e., hemophiliacs)—were much the same cross-nationally (with important exceptions, to be noted below). Both countries' blood systems were largely self-governing by medical elites chosen from their own ranks, and medical elites dominated the system overall. Blood bankers in both countries were organizationally highly invested in the cultivation and care of blood donors. And as blood services metamorphosed from a localized, artisanal activity into a multimillion-dollar business, these actors confronted similar contradictions.

Conflicts and Contradictions Within the Field

Contradiction in the logics applied to human blood emerged almost simultaneously with recognition of its therapeutic potential, increasing exponentially as discovery of blood's multiple properties and uses in medicine raised its value to consumers, both doctors and patients. Every country with a medical system sufficiently advanced to routinely use human blood in medical practice confronted the questions of whether blood donation should be paid or voluntary and of whether blood systems should or should not be "nonprofit." These were not trivial issues, since ensuring a reliable supply of the essential raw material (whole blood), organizing its distribution across space and time and, eventually, scaling up the manufacture of blood products (fractionation) were expensive propositions. Over time, France settled on

---

[5] Report on the Activity of the Committee on Energy and Commerce for the 103d Cong., 1st Sess. 1994: 152ff.

the logic of the gift embodied in (1) a countrywide network of independent nonprofit blood centers (including a small number engaged in fractionation) and (2) a politically powerful complex of beliefs (symbolic constructions) centered on the idea not only of blood donation itself as voluntary (a gift) but also an entire institution—its practices and its beliefs—grounded in altruism. With the pharmaceuticalization of blood, pressures from within the French government to develop an independent (i.e., nationally self-reliant) and internationally competitive pharmaceutical manufacturing sector, and EU pressures to regulate blood in the same category as pharmaceutical drugs, the contradictions between theory (the mythology of a voluntary nonprofit system) and practice (e.g., juggling finances to avoid bankruptcy) became intense. In 1991, those contradictions—heretofore relatively well hidden— became visible in the public arena, creating institutional waves within and well beyond the healthcare system.

Beginning in the mid-1940s and through the 1960s, the United States confronted these same contradictions on multiple levels and in multiple institutional contexts, not only within the blood system itself but also in regulatory bodies, in Congress, and in the courts with outcomes that were inconsistent. Within a few years of one another, courts ruled—on the one hand—that blood transfusion was a service, not a sale, while the Federal Trade Commission ruled—on the other hand—that transactions in human blood were governed by the laws of the market. As this inconsistency demonstrates, although contradictions between ideas and practices (institutional rules and relational structures) treating blood as a commodity and as a gift existed in the United States, there was no overriding system of beliefs governing their resolution. In the early 1970s, under pressure in part from Richard Titmuss's devastating attack on what he characterized as the dangers of the U.S. blood system to human health (Titmuss [1970] 1997), a form of resolution was devised creating two systems: one for the manufacture of blood products dependent on paid donations and openly market based and for profit; the other for transactions in whole blood, nonprofit, and based on voluntary donations. Contradictory logics were rendered invisible to the public by segregating their operations into separate, complementary, and noncompeting, bounded institutions occupying different social spaces. Confronted by the common threat in the early 1980s of HIV in the blood supply, the impulse of these two institutions was not to engage in mutual finger-pointing but to join forces to avert legal liability, a concern that brought noncommercial and commercial blood bankers together, overriding both long-standing institutional antagonisms and also contradictory institutional logics.[6]

Strategic Mobilization

Beliefs and practices—the cultural schemas that frame actions as good or evil, legitimate or illegitimate, and the rules and relationships that embody those schemas—are in practice inseparable and exercise their influence simultaneously (Beckert 2010). It is only for analytic purposes—to identify the differences in key actors' access to cultural and material resources that led to destabilization/mobilization in one case and not in the other—that we describe these elements separately, beginning with cultural schemas. In keeping with the work of Swidler (1986), Benford and Snow (2000) and others, we distinguish between cultural schemas as *resources*—a "'tool kit' of symbols, stories, rituals, and world-views, which people [i.e., interested actors including but not limited to social movement entrepreneurs] may use in varying configurations to solve different kinds of problems" (Swidler 1986:273) and the "collective action frames" that movement actors draw on to mobilize potential constituents and allies. Cultural schemas are at one and the same time a highly flexible resource, a lens, and a key to strategic mobilization.

Gifts, Commodities, and the Technological Imperative

On the surface, the starkest difference between France and the United States was the moral outrage and sense of profound betrayal that followed the discovery of contamination of the blood supply in France. What was interpreted in the United States—reflected most clearly in the Dingell hearings—as a failure of technological regulation, to be corrected by better regulation, was in France a breach of what were believed to be impenetrable moral boundaries. At stake was less the contamination itself—accidental contamination, however lethal, would not have aroused comparable outrage—but what was

---

[6] Although the noncommercial (whole blood) and commercial (blood products) systems were formally segregated, the boundary was, in reality, extremely fuzzy, as the work of Gilbert Gaul (1989a–e) and Douglas Starr (2002) make clear.

framed by interested actors of all stripes as "the eruption of market logic into a matter of life and death" (Casteret 1992:58). Journalists (e.g., Casteret, Greilsamer) but equally scholars (Hermitte, Chauveau, Fillion) portrayed the blood affair as the outcome of an inherent contradiction between France's industrial (encompassing technological and scientific) ambition and its devotion to humanistic values (encompassing human dignity and public health). Hermitte proposed the concept of "*délinquence technologique*"—technological delinquency—as a quasi-legal category to describe "indifference" of industrialists (viz. Garretta) to scientific and technological risks (1996:342). Society owed a moral debt to hemophiliacs and other "victims of progress" from which the state and industrialists profited (Hermitte 1996:329).

As Rabinow observes, "the science, the technology [of transfusion], and much of the blood circulated across national borders, across oceans. The institutions and their associated cultures and symbols did not" (1999:74). Appadurai defines a commodity as "anything intended for exchange" and, following his approach, it is useful to think of blood as a "thing" that moves in and out of the commodity state and of its commodification as a phase in the social life of blood. French and American publics had quite different normative perspectives on how that movement should be governed: "The flow of commodities in any given situation is a shifting compromise between socially regulated paths and competitively inspired diversions" (Appadurai 1986:17). From the French perspective, commodification of blood was an immoral diversion from the socially regulated and approved path of blood— juridically "*hors du commerce*" in all its phases from supplier to consumer. From the U.S. perspective, the trajectory of blood was uneven and largely invisible, its status as a commodity uncertain but not of central moral concern. Even when made visible (e.g., by Gilbert Gaul in the *Philadelphia Inquirer*), the knowledge that there was big money in blood may have caught the attention of Congress but hardly caused a ripple in the public sphere. High-tech medicine was expected to cost money.

A recent wave of comparative work has drawn attention to clashing European and American worldviews of science, technology, and the commodification of life. Parthasarathy describes the 1980 *Diamond v. Chakrabarty* case when "the United States . . . opened its doors wide to life-form patentability, famously allowing patents 'on anything under the sun made by man'" (2017:2), dismissing ethical and socioeconomic considerations that Europeans take seriously. Fourcade quotes a French environmental activist in an oil spill case: "I, for one, firmly believe that putting a price on something that has no price, and I think specifically of ecological damage, is by nature debasing" (2011:1767). Rabinow recounts the conflict with their American counterparts but also among French scientists themselves over the ownership and price of "French DNA" (1999). These vignettes are relevant to our story on multiple levels. First (with the partial exception of Rabinow), this work has ignored the central role of the blood affair *as it was construed in France* in shaping later European and French perspectives privileging the moral dimension over the scientific/technological dimension of biotechnological questions and events (see in addition to the contributions cited above, Jasanoff 2005, Vogel 2012). Although the first inklings of the precautionary principle grew from environmental concerns, it was the blood affair that transformed biotechnology into a clear and present danger highly visible to publics and policymakers on the European continent but almost imperceptible in the United States.[7]

Vocabularies of pollution—the threat posed by intrusion of the profane into sacred space—are hardly new and were equally available to actors on both sides of the Atlantic (as were vocabularies privileging the advance of science and technology). But the powerful resonance of pollution vocabularies in France—especially when the profane took a monetary form—has been well documented (Rabinow 1999, Lamont 1992, 2000, Lamont and Thévenot 2000, Fourcade 2011). Parthasarathy traces to the sixteenth century a uniquely European concern with the "moral" dimension of patents on innovative technology and the demand for government intervention to ensure protection of the public interest against the greedy market (2017:22ff.). Fourcade cites Tocqueville to argue that historically "aristocratic" societies (e.g., France) are particularly resistant to the leveling effect of money that reduces all "things" to "a single metric of worth" (2011:1729).[8] The ongoing power of these beliefs (and their relative absence in the United States) was clear (as Fourcade also observes) in

---

[7] In his memoir of life as a member of several French health ministerial cabinets, Didier Tabuteau observed that "independent developments in environmental and public health rights converged in 1992 under the pressure of events. Reform of the [French] blood transfusion system precipitated dramatically by the affair of the contaminated blood coincided with the final debate on ratification of the treaty of Maastricht [that formalized the precautionary principle in Europe]" (2006:46). A stark and very current example of the difference in French and American perspectives on biotechnology and the commodification of life are the legal restrictions on surrogacy and other reproductive technologies in France as compared with the increasing "financialization" of fertility in the United States (Bruch et al. 2020, Borsa and Bruch 2022).

[8] Alexander dates the demonization of capitalism and the market from the work of radical British political economists in the early nineteenth century, subsequently amplified (and popularized) by Marx (2006:25).

Lamont's (1992, 2000) extended interviews with middle- and working-class French and American men and in a series of comparative essays edited by Lamont and Thévenot (2000). French respondents were uniformly uncomfortable with putting a monetary value on moral worth, Americans far less so. By the early 1990s, with the dramatic successes of *bio*technology—the technologization of the human—and its even more dramatic (in French eyes) failures—intellectual, policy, and public anxiety about health, safety, and environmental risks imposed by greedy corporations and industrially ambitious states had become acute.

The important difference between France and the United States was less in scientific uncertainty about biotechnological risk than in how those risks were framed and resolved—in the United States as a morally neutral question to be answered by some form of risk-benefit analysis (by the IOM, for example, in their retrospective examination of the blood affair), in France as a morally fraught question in which—after the blood affair and informed by that experience—risks to human dignity and integrity overrode expected benefits, especially if those benefits were proclaimed by financially interested parties.

Actors, Allies, Opponents, and Opportunities

In both countries actors in the blood field were embedded in complex networks of internal and external relationships with suppliers (donors), blood bankers (split in the United States between organized collectors of the raw material [whole blood] and pharmaceutical manufacturers of blood products), blood recipients (of whom only hemophiliacs were organized in both countries), state administrators and regulators, other political actors, lawyers, and journalists. In a causal analysis of U.S. blood policies, Healy argued that the relative scarcity of suppliers (donors) led whole blood bankers to make decisions protective of donor interests while manufacturers that used paid donors and had no dearth of suppliers were more concerned with protecting their relatively rare customers. He neglected both blood bankers' and manufacturers' extreme sensitivity to the threat of legal liability, as much concerned with protection of their industry as with protection of their donors. The French system where blood was collected from unpaid donors irrespective of its destination as whole blood or blood products offered no incentive for French fractionators to protect consumers corresponding to the incentive for manufacturers in the United States: donors were the undisputed Gods of the French system.

Our interest is less in causal analysis and more in how embedded interests and power relationships (interdependencies) led to different retrospective reconstructions of events that happened in the early 1980s (e.g., attributions of scientific knowledge and/or uncertainty) by French and American authorities, lawyers, and journalists, and to these actors' different incentives for and against the amplification of crisis. The basic facts of scientific knowledge, blood contamination, and massive HIV infection of hemophiliacs and transfusees were the same in both countries, as we have noted. What was different was the relative power of various organizational actors to mobilize political connections and resources for and against the amplification of contamination and infection into political crisis. Our argument is that the institutional forces lined up *against* amplification were substantially more powerful in the United States than in France.[9]

France experienced the blood affair as a massive betrayal by the state of its fundamental obligation to ensure the security of its people. This reading did not spring up overnight or unaided, nor was the readily available vocabulary of struggle between sacred and profane values sufficient on its own to account for the blood crisis. Crisis was socially produced by the mobilization of affected communities but also—and equally important—by political opportunities for mobilization present in France but delayed, nonexistent, or closed off in the United States.

Both France and the United States had patient organizations of hemophiliacs that preexisted AIDS and served—with more or less delay and to varying degrees—as "mobilizing structures" bringing hemophiliacs with AIDS together and advocating on their behalf. Both countries saw the emergence of "radical flank" militant hemophiliac groups to contest what many hemophiliacs perceived not only as the laggard behavior of their traditional associations but also as these associations' complaisance with the state and (in the United States) with manufacturers of blood products (in France the first radical flank quickly acquired a second even more radical flank). Despite these similarities, the organizational and associational landscapes that

---

[9] This implies that in the absence of those powerful forces there would have been a blood crisis in the United States. Not necessarily. There were other differences between the two countries that may also have increased the relative probability of crisis in France: less fear among hemophiliacs of coming forward, greater suspicion of technology and its purveyors, and greater suspicion of market-based values.

confronted affected persons in the two countries as well as the constellation of incentives and opportunities for mobilization, let alone the production of political crisis, were entirely different, almost the inverse of one another. First, the threat of stigma and discrimination against persons with AIDS had been officially and publicly disowned in France by 1987, at least six years earlier than in the United States. Second, militant hemophiliacs (and transfusees) in France rapidly acquired vocal and influential allies not only in the press but also among newly organized gays; and, at least equally influential if more discreet, in the French prosecutorial system tasked with investigating their cases as *parties civiles* against the CNTS and other targets. Internal competition within the fields *both* of journalists *and* of AIDS organizations amplified these actors' incentives for mobilization and crisis amplification. Third, France's centralization—political, cultural, and geographic—along with its hierarchical political structure made it relatively easy (compared with the United States) for militants to concentrate their forces against the state as culprit rather than taking on a more fragmented array of blood banks and blood bankers. Finally, many of the obstacles that confronted hemophiliacs and transfused patients in the United States—AIDS-related stigma, powerful gay rights organizations already on the scene, phalanxes of lawyers primed to appear on behalf of blood banks and blood product manufacturers, and an easily mobilized blood system and pharmaceutical constituency prepared to counter assaults on the powerful FDA—simply did not exist or existed to a much lesser degree in France.

French activists were united in identifying the principal threat to the hemophiliac community as AIDS. American hemophiliacs—bombarded by stories in the press and on TV of children vilified and kept out of school, families menaced, and houses torched—saw the principal threat as AIDS-associated stigma and discrimination. It was not until the early 1990s after the (relatively) gay friendly Clinton administration had come to power and begun to shift the AIDS narrative away from the moralizing tone taken by prior Republican administrations that hemophiliacs in the United States came out of hiding and publicly organized on behalf of their community. In France, once sickness and death among its members became visible to the AFH in the mid-1980s, its leaders quietly approached the minister of health to ask for monetary relief. The AFH's "radical flank," whose leader wrote to members of Parliament and talked to journalists, was formed at about the same time; their narrative of state dissimulation and betrayal was rapidly diffused. There was *no organized pushback* by blood bankers to counter these efforts (if the blood bankers even knew about them) or to establish a different narrative. French blood banking was highly fragmented as it was in the United States, but unlike the United States, there were no professional organizations to represent blood bankers' interests nor was there anything comparable to the powerful American Red Cross responsible for collecting one-half of the U.S. blood supply. France's largest blood-banking groups were highly competitive with one another; the nearest they had to a representative body was the Commission Consultative de Transfusion Sanguine (CCTS). France's blood bankers had nothing comparable to the American Association of Blood Banks (AABB), the Council of Community Blood Centers (CCBC), the American Blood Resources Association (ABRA), and the Red Cross, each organization with its staff of lawyers to represent them before the courts, the Congress, and the executive branch. Alerted by the CDC in January 1983, these organizations immediately recognized their potential legal liability and convened to align their interests and establish an agreed-upon exculpatory narrative.[10] A further striking element of the American case was the routine presence of representatives from gay organizations at meetings called by U.S. official bodies to address blood supply questions. Gay men had been excellent blood donors (accounting for 15–25% of donations, depending on location), and they were immediately implicated as potential sources of contamination. Their cooperation in actions to protect the blood supply was heavily solicited by health officials and blood bankers, who wanted to protect their relationship with these excellent donors.[11]

Despite the French dedication to a voluntary blood system (both for whole blood and for blood products) and the presence throughout the country of organized blood donors with excellent political connections, the French donor association was not represented in the Garretta trial and proved largely ineffective as an advocate for French blood banks.[12] French victims had engaged the state prosecutorial system on their behalf well before the crisis rupture of 1991 both as investigator of the facts and eventually as prosecutor.

[10] This narrative became the "standard of care" on which judges based their decisions in court cases brought against blood bankers by hemophiliacs and transfusees, leading to their dismissal in the majority of instances.

[11] Blood bankers in both countries were extremely reluctant to ask questions about sexual practices that might offend their donors. But only in the United States were gays both specifically identified as "good" donors and organized to protect their interests against what they interpreted as discrimination.

[12] Before the blood crisis, donor organization members had played a significant role in the process of blood donation, removing needles, applying bandages, and the like. Reform of the blood system resulted in their exclusion with these roles assumed by hospital personnel (Chauveau 2011:232).

At the Garretta trial, although the accused had their individual lawyers, blood banks as organizations—even the CNTS—had no legal representation. "Victims" were represented by the state. French blood bankers had no legal levers to smother the crisis before it emerged comparable to those available to their American counterparts. By the time the French state actively intervened under Kouchner to reorganize the blood system, blood bankers had been thoroughly discredited in court and by the press, and bankers and their allies (i.e., the donor association) had very little countervailing power. In the United States, as we have described in detail in Chapter 3, blood banks, manufacturers, and the Red Cross were able to use their internal networks, their external political connections (with the FDA, with other members of government, with gay rights organizations, with the press[13]), and the legal system to sustain their preferred narrative of reassurance and control, to avoid public accountability, and to prevent an eruption of crisis into the public sphere.

Gay rights organizations were of critical importance in shaping the organizational landscape confronted by hemophiliacs and transfusees. Their roles in the two countries could hardly have been more different. By the early 1980s in France, any semblance of a politically engaged gay rights movement had disappeared, and—unlike in the United States—gays had no role in HIV/AIDS blood policymaking. In neither country were blood bankers enthusiastic about interrogating potential donors about their sexual behavior, and in both countries gays interpreted screening questions as discrimination, but only in the United States did gay rights organizations align with blood bankers in organized opposition to AIDS-related screening. In France, all the mainstream political parties moved against Le Pen's efforts to stigmatize and quarantine gays; in the United States, Republican Jesse Helms and his allies in Congress seized upon every opportunity, including threats to the blood supply, to regulate and criminalize gay blood donation. Not only were gay organizations aligned with blood bankers in the United States to oppose what they interpreted as discrimination against gay blood donors, but they

---

[13] A *Philadelphia Inquirer* reporter told us that his editor was visited by an official from the Red Cross aiming to suppress articles on blood banking and HIV/blood contamination. Although the official was unsuccessful in this case, this anecdote demonstrates how far blood bankers were willing to go in their effort to stay under the public radar. Although this is mere speculation, it seems unlikely that the *Inquirer* was the only newspaper visited by the Red Cross, and it is possible that other newspaper editors were more amenable to pressure from this highly prestigious organization. It is worth noting that the Red Cross was highly successful in obtaining protective orders from judges such that "thousands of Red Cross documents were sealed from the public, press, and plaintiff attorneys" (Reitman 1996:74–75).

also shared with Democratic politicians and activists the desire to avoid giving political opportunities for gay-bashing to Helms and Republicans. The production of a political crisis around blood was the last thing these actors wanted.

The political landscape for French gay activists in the late 1980s was almost exactly the opposite. Act Up-Paris was formed in the late 1980s. AIDES was "the" establishment association already in the field. It presented itself not as pro-gay but as anti-AIDS and until that point had occupied almost all the relevant associational space. The blood affair presented an ideal opportunity for this new, militant, small group of openly gay activists to put itself on the map. Amplification of crisis was entirely in its interests. Act Up-Paris rapidly took up the cause of blood contamination "victims" (principally hemophiliacs) *against* blood bankers and the "murderous" state, taking every opportunity for open public demonstration of its righteous wrath. The 1992 Garretta trial was just such an opportunity, and Act Up-Paris took full advantage of it, instrumentalizing the visibility of hemophiliacs as a popular cause to assert its own organizational presence and power in France's AIDS landscape at the time.

Rupture

The stage for transformation of health catastrophe into political crisis was set in France: first, by the presence of publicly unacknowledged contradictions in the institutional logics that governed transactions in human blood; second, by processes of strategic mobilization that brought those contradictions into the public sphere; and third, by a set of beliefs that labeled those contradictions as immoral and unacceptable. We have borrowed from Aldon Morris's (1993) description of civil rights movement tactics in Birmingham, Alabama, in 1963 to label events preceding the moment of rupture in the spring of 1991 as "strategic mobilization." The goal of movement actions in the Birmingham case—shutting down the town's business district through coordinated social protest—was to generate a crisis of such magnitude that national and local white establishments would have no option but to capitulate. The goals of French advocates for HIV/blood victims in 1987–1991 may have been less calculated, but the combination of increasingly bellicose threats of public exposure, strategic leaks of damning information to the press, recruitment of key allies, and street protests by AIDS activists had all the elements of strategic mobilization, generating a crisis that did, indeed, force the government to capitulate. We argue that while contradictions within the blood field were present in the United States, the other two necessary conditions were absent. First, opportunities for strategic mobilization in the United States were limited both by hemophiliacs' initial (understandable) reluctance to come forward and (more important) by an array of networked and mobilized institutional and political actors within and external to the blood field for whom advocating on behalf of hemophiliacs was contrary to their interests. Second, contamination of the blood supply was framed in the United States as a technological/scientific/medical problem, not a moral problem, so no profound moral beliefs were engaged.

Paradoxes and Anomalies

In his authoritative study of French public bureaucracy, Michel Crozier described France as "a centralized power that has become paralyzed because of its omnipotence and its concomitant isolation" (1964:234). Nowhere has this paralysis been more evident than in the domain of public health (Nathanson 2007). Nathanson attributed France's historic weakness in this domain to five factors, three of which are central to the present case: first, "the perception of the state as the sole legitimate policy actor"; second, a "corresponding underdevelopment of activism by ordinary people"; third, "the power of France's medical practitioners to shape health-related public policies to suit their professional interests" (2007:209).[14] Despite this long history of "delayed or ineffective public health action" (documented in Nathanson's book *Disease Prevention as Social Change*), "confronted by extraordinary circumstances, that is, crises with the real or imagined potential for political damage to the state, the French government has been quite capable of rapid action" (2007:211).

The rapid government actions that followed Casteret's publication in *L'Événement du jeudi* in the spring of 1991 were precipitated by just such an extraordinary circumstance. The health crisis itself had long passed. It was the *political crisis* that demanded action.

[14] The other two factors were "the popular and political assumption of state omnipotence" and "a powerful, persistent, and perhaps surprising strain of antistatism." The first factor is subsumed by the "state as sole legitimate policy actor"; "antistatism" played a minimal role in the blood affair.

We have advanced what we believe to be a widely applicable framework to specify the conditions under which contradictions within an institutional field do or do not morph into political crises. These processes are contingent, however, with both crisis amplification and response playing out in variable historical and political landscapes that shape their specific contours. First, although the modes of collective action employed by French hemophiliacs and their allies were novel in the French context, their insistence on targeting the state as, indeed, "the sole legitimate policy actor" was entirely consistent with French history and practice: "The French state is at the same time the owner of public health problems with the authority to create and influence the problem's public definition and the bearer of political responsibility for solving the problem. The state may also be accused of causing the problem by its neglect [as in the present case]" (Nathanson 2007:209). From the standpoint of newly politicized collective actors, appeal to the state was the "natural course" (Haas 1992:64). Second, and equally important in enabling rapid state action in response to the blood crisis, was the total discrediting of medical authority. Vilified in the press and by their patients, brought to public account in a Paris court, physicians lost (at least temporarily) their traditional power to shape health policy. (Ironically, among those who took advantage of the political opportunities created by this loss of authority were several prominent physician-politicians.)

The account of Francis Kelsey and the FDA with which Monica Prasad opens *The Land of Too Much* (described in Chapter 1) is intended to make the point that traditional portrayals of the United States as a "weak state" are simply wrong: the United States is, in fact, a very strong state; its power is employed in ways not captured by the European idea of centralized political and territorial power. Nathanson made a similar argument in *Disease Prevention as Social Change* (2007) that the United States was not so much a weak state as one that departed from the European model in both the style and circumstances in which its power was deployed. The thalidomide story broke in the early 1960s. In light of the FDA's celebrated actions then, the absence of regulatory action when it came to blood is striking. We have argued in Chapter 4 and above that the FDA was both embedded in and protected by "a networked congeries of audiences" (Eyal 2019:135) that acted in the 1980s blood case both to inhibit regulatory action and to insulate the agency from the consequences of inaction.

Historically, a critical difference between France and the United States has been the fact that the United States has many more strings to its bow, strings that do not depend on the action or inaction of the central state—more actors outside the state eager to swing their weight in public policy arenas and more arenas where that weight can make a difference. In his analysis of "political opportunity structures and political protest," Kitschelt placed France and the United States at opposite poles: the French political system "closed" to protest demands with high capacity to "ward off threats to the implementation of policies" (1986:66); the United States "open" to demands but with weak capacity for implementation. And so, among the many paradoxes of the blood story are, *first*, the early activism of French hemophiliacs as compared with the United States and the critical part played by journalists and militant gays in shaping, publicizing, and politicizing the French crisis narrative; *second*, the *inability* of the French state to "ward off" the threat these actions posed; and *finally*, the eventual adoption of militants' demands in the form of policy innovation. In this rare case political "openness"—forced by the processes of crisis production we have described—and political "capacity" converged (Kitschelt 1986:67).

In the U.S. civil society action in the AIDS arena was dominated by gay men; their role in the blood story was as suppliers reacting against discrimination in the marketplace of blood, not as supporters of consumer-friendly regulation, nor did they model solidarity with other victims of HIV as did AIDES in France. As we have argued earlier, this dominance left little space or place in the public sphere for militant hemophiliacs to make their case. Political opportunities were blocked as well by a largely disinterested press, a distracted national administration, and a blood system well positioned to protect its interests from attack by unfortunate consumers (or intrusive government regulators).

Conclusion

The *critical* difference that produced a political crisis in France and its absence in the United States was not in beliefs and institutions but in the networks of relationships that surrounded each set of actors in the blood field and in which they were embedded. These relationships empowered strategic mobilization of hemophiliacs and their allies in France and blocked mobilization in the United States. *In France*, competitive relationships within the media and among AIDS associations drove amplification of the crisis; relationship ties among blood bankers and of blood bankers with politicians and officials fell apart under threat of exposure. *In the United States*, close ties among blood bankers and of blood bankers with key regulatory officials led them—in sharp contrast to their French counterparts—to identify the threat to their "stable business" early on and to rapidly close ranks against exposure in the courts (and possibly in the media as well). The AIDS field in the United States was already in the early 1980s dominated by organized gay men leaving little associational space for hemophiliacs; further, gay men were important blood suppliers, and their interests in pushing back against what was perceived as discrimination in blood donation aligned with those of blood bankers in maintaining the blood supply. Finally, relationship ties between organized gays and Democratic politicians may have played a role as well in deflecting the latter's attention away from the AIDS/blood connection.

In their 1999 review article, Clemens and Cook made a strong argument for the importance of social network ties in maintaining institutional stability: "Dense network ties . . . establish the conditions for maintaining order and punishing defectors from institutional arrangements" (Clemens and Cook 1999:451). Our comparative work supports this argument but also points to the complex role of network ties in challenging stability as well as maintaining it.

10

Conclusion

Crisis and Change

We close this book with three sets of reflections: first, on the ongoing ripples from the blood scandal in France; second, on the reach of our conceptual framework; and third, on the contingent politics of epidemics.

Ripples in France

Sewell theorizes "historical events" as occurrences that "change the course of history": "an occurrence only becomes a historical event, in the sense in which [Sewell uses] the term, when it touches off a chain of occurrences that durably transforms previous structures and practices" (1996:843). This transformative process entails (as specified by Sewell) spread of the initial rupture (or crisis) from its starting point to other locations and structures (i.e., crisis amplification) as well as significant changes in the structures themselves (beliefs, networks, modes of power). Whether or not any given "occurrence" qualifies as an event (i.e., whether structures have or have not been durably transformed) is a post hoc judgement, made with some confidence when dealing with an event that occurred over 200 years ago and whose consequences have been fixed for some time (Sewell's example is the taking of the Bastille), more tentatively when the consequences of a rupture have only recently begun to appear. We argue that the *affaire du sang* qualifies not only as a rupture but also as an "event" in Sewell's sense of a transformation of structures.

The consequences of the blood scandal in France did not end with the deaths and personal and family tragedies caused by toxic blood or with the unleashing of the media, the resignation of politicians, and proceedings before the Cour de justice de la République that followed the revelations of *L'Événement du jeudi* in 1991. The scandal triggered a profound restructuring of French public health to the point where even the management of

The Social Production of Crisis. Constance A. Nathanson and Henri Bergeron, Oxford University Press.
© Oxford University Press 2023. DOI: 10.1093/oso/9780197682487.003.0010

the COVID-19 crisis drew in part on this heritage. The political and policy consequences of the blood scandal have been threefold: (1) the construction of a large body of policies and organizational structures around the concept of "*sécurité sanitaire*" that have in the years following the blood crisis absorbed "public health" in France; (2) a deliberate fostering of the rights of patients and users of healthcare as a field of practice; and (3) reinforcement of the state's (and of the central government's) quasi-monopolistic role in health-crisis management. The goal of these policies has been to restore public confidence in the French state's traditional role as the benevolent guardian of its citizens, confidence profoundly shaken by the scandal of toxic blood.

The first steps in this project of restoration were the invention of *sécurité sanitaire* and the construction of a distinct and clearly identified political and policy space around this concept (Alam 2010).[1] Over time, this space became associated with key underlying principles, including preventing conflicts of interest in regulatory matters (i.e., the fox guarding the henhouse) and, perhaps of most significance, the precautionary principle. Adoption of this principle reflected a substantial shift in the French conception of risk, above all in the attribution of responsibility for "therapeutic accidents." "The fact of having acted on the basis of current knowledge (scientific, technical, social) is not sufficient to relieve individuals of responsibility for decisions or acts that result in harm" (Lascoumes 1996:365).[2] In 2005, the precautionary principle was written into the French Constitution, an act attributable at least in part to continuing fallout from the *affaire du sang*.

Beyond the development of organizing principles, the social and policy space represented by *sécurité sanitaire* was populated by a number of independent agencies, two in direct response to the toxic blood scandal: the French Blood Agency (Agence Française du Sang) and the Medicines Agency (Agence du Médicament) (Nathanson and Bergeron 2017).[3] These agencies were conceived as bureaucratic responses charged with limiting the risk that new crises and scandals would surface. If officially these agencies were intended to reinforce the domain of public health, in fact their creation was

---

[1] *Sécurité sanitaire* is literally translated "health security" but the phrase has a far more muscular connotation in French than in English, invoking historical and contemporary references to government intervention on behalf of public order and public welfare. We leave it in the original French.

[2] This latter principle is what is known in Anglo-Saxon jurisprudence as "strict liability."

[3] The emergence of these agencies also benefited from the diffusion of "new public management," a concept promoting principles of transparency, independent expertise, and the separation of analysis of risk from risk management, an organizational form and set of institutional and management principles that circulated internationally (Benamouzig and Besançon 2005, Alam and Godard 2007).

perceived as extending the reach of *sécurité sanitaire* to the point that subse-quent governments felt it necessary to pass a law (law "about public health," passed on August 9, 2004) affirming that *sécurité sanitaire* was not ALL of public health (Bergeron and Nathanson 2014).

The law on "the right of patients and the quality of the healthcare system" was passed on March 4, 2002, over ten years after the toxic blood scandal. But the intellectual project for the promotion of patient rights both individually and collectively was initiated in 1989 under the health ministry of Claude Evin (FNA, Box 910611-1 [CAB 506], April 12, 1989). This law was not only a response to patient and allied mobilization around HIV (hemophiliacs, transfusees, and gay men) but also equally intended as a measure to repair the erosion of trust between health authorities and citizens (Bergeron 2007, 2013). The social movements that arose in response to the AIDS epidemic had publicly challenged all established authorities—economic, political, ad-ministrative, and, in particular, scientific—in a fashion previously unheard of in French health politics (Buton 2005). At one and the same time the su-periority of scientific discourse was contested (Callon et al. 2001) and legit-imacy asserted for the contribution of "lay experts" to processes hitherto dominated by credentialed "scientists" (Benamouzig and Besançon 2005). It was in this context that the French conception of "*démocratie sanitaire*" (health democracy) conceived as complementary to "*démocratie sociale*" (social democracy) was introduced.

The third policy outcome of the blood scandal was the state's assertion of a baronial role in the domain of public health comparable to its traditional role in the maintenance of national security and public order.[4] Protection of its citizens had long been central to the French idea of the state. The blood affair precipitated a marked expansion of this role: health crises were newly identified as threats to the nation-state compelling a state-level response. To the state's human enemies (external and internal) were now added "epidemics, poverty, [and] environmental degradation," calling for new forms of contention (Borraz and Gilbert 2008:337). Key elements of this role were, first, the concentration of funds, personnel, and expertise in multiple new agencies that embodied (literally in their titles and also in their intent) the notion of *sécurité sanitaire*; and, second, an unprecedented increase and

---

[4] The role of the state in promoting and organizing "health and hygiene" (i.e., public health) for its "citizen-patients" was a guiding principle of the French Revolution (Nathanson 2007:31). Not until the *affaire du sang* in 1992, over 200 years later, did this principle gain serious traction.

expansion in the power of the state to manage (what it defined as) public health crises (Tabuteau 2007).

There continue to be continuities in the closed, highly centralized decision processes characteristic of the French state (see, e.g., Kitschelt 1986). Since at least 1954 public health laws—however shaped by the politics of the moment—have been elaborated and powered through Parliament by entrepreneurial health ministers and their immediate (often intimate) colleagues and associates (Bergeron and Castel 2014:389). The management of the COVID-19 crisis bears all the marks of this approach, led almost entirely by elites (Bergeron et al. 2020). Important decisions were made by a very small number of highly placed individuals: the president of the Republic, his prime minister, the health minister, and a scientific council, the latter an ad hoc creation envisioned by no prior law or plan, its composition highly restricted and covered by the French equivalent of the (British) Official Secrets Act. The advantage of this formation from the government's perspective was to maximize its capacity for autonomous and unconstrained decision-making (Bergeron et al. 2020). In this state-centric and hyper-centralized approach to crisis management, local authorities and intermediate bodies played a distinctly secondary role as little more than channels of information whose perspectives and actions were, if not forbidden, at the very least discouraged (Bergeron et al. 2020). The contrast with fragmented decision processes in the United States can hardly be overstated.

Conceptual Reach

We have argued that our conceptual framework has application beyond the specific case that led to its development. Here we briefly reprise that framework and examine other public health events in its light with the dual aims of assessing its value and pointing to new directions for research and theory. Our framework has three elements: first, underlying contradictions in the institutional logics that animate an important "field" of action; second, a process of strategic mobilization that renders these contradictions visible in the public sphere; and third, cultural beliefs that frame those contradictions as immoral and unacceptable. We believe that all three of these elements are necessary to the production of political crisis and that absent any one of them, a political crisis is unlikely to emerge.

Although health events in the United States are often politicized (smoking, HIV, and COVID-19 are obvious recent examples), they rarely become crises that threaten existing political institutions. President Trump was not twice impeached because he mismanaged the coronavirus epidemic. We compare two events we have alluded to earlier—the 1970s blood scare triggered by Richard Titmuss's book *The Gift Relationship* and passage of the Ryan White Act triggered by mobilization around HIV—the first a disturbance without a crisis, the second an outcome of publicly proclaimed crisis—to illustrate how our framework might contribute to the analysis of these events and to an understanding of the contingencies imposed by their political setting.

Contradictions within the U.S. blood system arose simultaneously with the commodification and commercialization of blood and blood products as stated in the previous chapter. The threat of hepatitis was well known to specialists in the field, noted in 1960s congressional hearings and in a 1970 report from the National Academy of Sciences, and brought to the attention of the FDA, the AFL-CIO, the American Red Cross, the AMA "and to congressmen in whose districts hepatitis had been publicized by the media" by concerned physicians and researchers (Starr 2002). Blood bankers felt threatened—"[they] recognized the danger of hepatitis, but worried more about their problems of supply, which, if the paid donor was eliminated, could escalate into a national crisis" (Starr 2002:220)—and critics of the blood system were initially dismissed. However, publication in 1971 of Titmuss's book denouncing flaws in the American system (including the high prevalence of hepatitis) as what happens when "critical areas of medicine [are subjected to] the laws of the marketplace" (cited in Starr 1998:227) "hit a public nerve." It generated scores of reviews in the news media and scholarly journals . . . waves of exposés appeared" (Starr 2002:228). *What this attention did not do was generate mobilization on the part of donors or consumers either to protest the stigmatization of paid blood donors (characterized as alcoholics, drug users, and criminals) or the dangers of exposure to toxic blood.* A task force "to look at new ways of managing the American blood supply" was formed within the Department of Health, Education, and Welfare (DHEW), several bills were introduced in Congress, the NIH and CDC conducted studies and—arguably the only significant outcome—DHEW made the executive decision to assign responsibility for regulation of the blood supply to the FDA. Meanwhile the Nixon administration turned reform of the blood system over to the system's warring blood banker factions: the American Red Cross, the American Association of Blood Banks, and the American Blood

Resources Association representing manufacturers. Unsurprisingly, these entities were unable to agree on a common framework for their actions, and what efforts they did make received little or no political support. Republicans in power had little interest in establishing a centralized blood system, and the Nixon administration quickly began to have other things on its mind. The reforms proposed dissolved before they got off the ground.

The critical differences between the hepatitis and HIV stories were, first, effective mobilization by people with AIDS and their political allies behind the legislation that became the Ryan White Act, and, second, framing this legislation as—at one and the same time—protection of innocent children and urban disaster relief—framings that effectively sidestepped the questions of "deservingness" that plague government forays into public healthcare funding in the United States.[5] The coalition behind the Ryan White Act was composed not only of gay organizations but also of 125 allied professional and civil society associations ranging from the PTA (Parent Teachers Association) to the AMA (American Medical Association). AIDS was framed certainly as an epidemic crisis but also as an urban healthcare crisis—hospitals and other health services on the verge of breakdown unable to cope with overwhelming demand, much as in the case of COVID-19. Political support for this legislation was reflected in its near unanimous passage by the U.S. Congress.

Both the 1970s blood scare around hepatitis and an out-of-control infectious disease epidemic exposed serious contradictions in the American healthcare system.[6] Yet only the latter produced a crisis sufficient to trigger significant social change: an unprecedented infusion of cash into the system itself and new templates for consumer participation both in healthcare management and in the evaluation of pharmaceutical drugs. The significant differences (our conceptual framework suggests, and we would argue) are, first, in "strategic mobilization" and, second, in framing. Fligstein and McAdam elaborate the useful concept of "incumbents": "Incumbents are those actors who wield disproportionate influence within a field and whose interests and views tend to be heavily reflected in [the field's] dominant organization" (2012:13). Even more to the point, fields often have "governance units" (Fligstein and McAdam's example is trade associations) that

---

[5] Protection of innocent children often seems like a sine qua non for government intervention in public health in the United States: anti-smoking campaigns used the same trope.

[6] "Toxic blood" encompasses both the hepatitis and the HIV-blood stories.

represent the field's most powerful incumbents and "can be expected to serve as defenders of the status quo and are a generally conservative force during periods of conflict" within the field (Fligstein and McAdam 2012:14). Trade associations "typically cultivate powerful allies in various state fields" (Fligstein and McAdam 2012:14). Incumbents in the American blood field were represented by powerful trade associations, they had close ties with one another and with federal authorities, their authority went almost entirely unchallenged until the mid-1990s, and even then the status quo was quickly restored. Whether the cause was hepatitis or HIV in the blood supply, opportunities for "strategic mobilization" against a monolithic industry, rich in wealth, power, and symbolism, were few and far between. In sharp contrast, early gay mobilization for healthcare to persons with HIV was joined by powerful "incumbents" in the healthcare field along with *their* "trade associations" (e.g., the American Hospital Association, the AMA) confronted with an epidemic hospitals and physicians lacked the resources to confront on their own. The status quo was unaffordable.

Yet even in this case of widely acknowledged breakdown in the healthcare *system*, arguments for the Ryan White Act were framed to deflect attention from systemic failure and toward the mysterious workings of fate and accident and the sufferings of infants and children. The divisiveness of this quintessentially American framing—the *deliberate* invoking of "innocent" victims to the implicit exclusion of the "guilty"—is highlighted by a comparison with French politicians' struggles over the framing of an equally unprecedented crisis-imposed financial outlay, the 1991 law compensating persons affected by HIV contamination of the blood supply. The principle underlying that law, invoked by government ministers and members of parliament alike, was that of *solidarité* with the victims of a catastrophe. Objections to the law were grounded not on its expansiveness—it made no distinction between infection by transfusion or blood products and extended coverage to widows, widowers, and children—but on its narrowness. The government was accused of "discrimination" against persons with hepatitis or other bloodborne infections and, indeed, against persons suffering from "therapeutic accidents" more generally.[7]

---

[7] In the United States we would probably translate "*accidents thérapeutique*" as "malpractice." This translation at one and the same time assumes a legal context and implies fault on the part of a physician. "Therapeutic accidents" does neither and corresponds much more closely to the French meaning.

The lessons drawn in France from the blood crisis were that modern technologies were dangerous and that the triumphs of modern medicine had a dark side in increased risk and potential for human suffering. In his introduction to a report he requested as minister of health on how his country should respond to *accidents thérapeutiques* Bernard Kouchner wrote: "Today we have discovered that the march of technical progress, from which we all benefit, does not marginalize risks; on the contrary, they are inherent in the beneficial activity itself. A society without risks does not exist. How those risks are managed is emblematic of society's social progress" (1992:11). Moral outrage fanned by mobilization in the public sphere created a political crisis that demanded a political response: protection against (or compensation for) human suffering orchestrated by the French state. The intensity of political crisis was reflected in the enormous scope of the state response we have described: the transformation of *santé publique* to *sécurité sanitaire*, the multiplication of public health agencies and expenditures on public health, embrace of the precautionary principle and, not least—although with considerable delay—the construction of an agency singularly devoted to protecting and compensating the victims of therapeutic accidents not through endless and often fruitless litigation but through expert adjudication.

Epidemic Politics, the Politics of Epidemics

Charles Rosenberg's 1989 article, "What Is an Epidemic?" written in the time of AIDS, has had a recent revival—and attracted trenchant if largely friendly critique—in the light of COVID-19.[8] Epidemics, Rosenberg proposed, have a characteristic "dramaturgic form": they "start at a moment in time, proceed on a stage limited in space and duration, follow a plot line of increasing and revelatory tension, move to a crisis of individual and collective character, then drift toward closure" (1989:2). At the same time, like crises more generally, "epidemics constitute an extraordinarily useful sampling device, at once found objects and natural experiments capable of illuminating fundamental patterns of social value and institutional practice" (Rosenberg 1989:2). It is on these intrasocietal and cross-national variations in "fundamental patterns" that Rosenberg's critics have focused, arguing from detailed

[8] See *Bulletin of the History of Medicine* 94, no. 4 (Winter 2020) for a series of articles critiquing and expanding Rosenberg's answers to the question posed by his title.

accounts of epidemic trajectories among marginalized communities and outside of Euro-American settings that epidemics do not always have clear beginnings and endings, that their visibility is not a defining characteristic but politically negotiated, that epidemics trigger opportunities and resilience as well as a search for culprits, and even that proclaiming an epidemic is itself a political act construing illness as a passing—and manageable—phenomena and allowing authorities to take credit for its end.

Nevertheless, even his critics have found Rosenberg's dramatic form a valuable thread around which to organize their epidemic narratives. A highly simplified version introduced our drama (within a drama) of AIDS and blood (Chapters 3 and 4). Rosenberg proposed three acts, Progressive Revelation (Act I), Managing Randomness (Act II), Negotiating Public Response (Act III), along with a less well defined fourth act in which the epidemic winds down. We use his framework to locate the political tensions specific to each "Act" in the AIDS/blood story as it played out in France and the United States. Political interests—calculations of gain and loss—shaped interpretations and actions at every stage and, ultimately, the epidemic's moral if not its biomedical trajectory.

Act I—Progressive Revelation

Reflecting on epidemics past, Rosenberg observed that "to admit the presence of an epidemic disease was to risk social dissolution" (Rosenberg 1989:4). "Dissolution" takes many forms. Blood bankers, faced with the specter of toxic blood and highly invested in the fragile chain from supplier to consumer that supported their industry, risked loss of suppliers at one end and consumers at the other end along with (in France) the mythology essential to its organization and (in the United States) their vaunted legal immunity. Relationships of physicians with patients (whether as donors or recipients) were threatened at every point as were the "normal lives" that hemophiliacs had come to confidently expect. The forms of threatened "dissolution" were specific to the HIV/blood affair, but the initial unenthusiastic response of authorities was classic: to proclaim "scientific" uncertainty and to kill the messenger—whether the messenger was a group of young importunate physicians (in France) or the CDC (in the United States). Epidemics do not "reveal" themselves; the "politics of visibility, concern, and ignorance" (Lachenal and Thomas 2020:13) have been a continuing thread throughout our narratives, reappearing every time a new document was "discovered" or quashed, a new actor dragged on the stage or an old one shunted off, or new interpretations of old data were voiced. Neither revelation nor concealment were confined to a single act.

Act II—Managing Randomness

This act might better be titled "managing non-randomness" since epidemic disease seldom strikes persons of all ages and stations alike. Random or not, what Rosenberg called "the dismaying arbitrariness" of epidemics—is hard to take, and once the threat can no longer be dismissed people seek explanations. In the Western canon "consolatory schemes have always centered on explaining the differential susceptibility of particular individuals" (Rosenberg 1989:5), in other words explaining why *someone else and not me* is more likely to get sick. Rosenberg pointed out that this "othering" or boundary construction very often took a moral turn, focusing on "belief in the connection of volition, responsibility, and susceptibility" (Rosenberg 1989:6). The experience of gays and hemophiliacs in the United States exemplify this pattern as we have shown, but the French case was different and more complicated. Randomness in the blood case was managed (arguably, it was embraced), and the epidemic among hemophiliacs "explained" not only by explicitly disavowing victim responsibility but also by publicly proclaiming the responsibility of the state. We suggest that "managing randomness" is highly contingent on what Lamont and Thévenot (2000) call "cultural repertoires of evaluation" and that in France the morality of "civic solidarity" overrode the morality of personal responsibility and drove the politics of public response to toxic blood.

Act III—Negotiating Public Response

Rosenberg made, but did not elaborate, the intriguing suggestion that "managing of response to epidemics could serve as a vehicle for social criticism as well as a rationale for social control" (Rosenberg 1989:6). The question follows, under what circumstances is "social criticism" more or less likely to emerge? Our conceptual framework is one answer to that question: the epidemic exposes morally unacceptable contradictions in the polity leading to widespread mobilization and rupture in the social fabric. A second set of circumstances that we have alluded to but not discussed in detail is *political opportunity*.[9] Weaknesses in the French blood system and in its public health services more generally were known to insiders well before the blood scandal (Murard and Zylberman 1996, Morelle 1996, Tabuteau 2006). Weaknesses in expertise and funding were compounded (and, of course exacerbated) by weaknesses in prestige within the French administrative hierarchy. Physicians as embodied in the relationship between doctor and patient were privileged and powerful, public health was "neglected and relegated to the second plan" (Tabuteau 2006:17). The blood crisis upended this structure, discrediting not only the doctors themselves but also their remedies—"revealed to be worse than the disease" (Tabuteau 2006:17). Peopled by enthusiastic young Turks recruited by health minister Bernard Kouchner and seizing opportunity in the midst of crisis, the French health cabinet in 1992 "embarked on reform of the organization of public health" (Tabuteau 2006:17) Far from drifting toward closure, as Rosenberg suggested, this program—encompassing social criticism and reform—continued as we have described above (and, of course, with varying success) long after the HIV/blood affair and even into later epidemics.

The United States is no stranger to the use of public health threats as opportunities for institution building. The current stature and power of the New York City Health Department owes much to cholera in the late nineteenth century and influenza in the early twentieth century and the CDC to the mid-twentieth-century threat of biological warfare (Fairchild et al. 2021). But epidemic plots are highly contingent on time and place and—as we have spelled out in some detail—the conditions that created rupture in the societal fabric and political opportunity for reform in France in the early 1990s did not exist in the United States. Perhaps the hardest to fathom is the absence of moral outrage at the massive deaths of hemophiliacs, a void that we mark but cannot fully explain.

In this country, protection against human suffering whether as a side effect of advances in medicine and technology or the structural violence of discrimination in all its forms is an ongoing contest between incumbents in power and those with the hardiness to challenge them, a dynamic that moral outrage seldom penetrates. Challengers do sometimes win but often at the

---

[9] The suggestion that epidemics may create individual and collective *opportunities* for growth and change is a principal theme of the articles collected in the *Bulletin of the History of Medicine* cited in the preceding footnote.

cost of having to prove their worthiness by showing they did not bring the suffering on themselves. In America, human suffering has no political privilege. Even highly visible and politicized health crises that generate nation-wide mobilization (e.g., HIV, Hurricane Katrina) are ultimately absorbed into the societal mainstream and pose little or no threat to the seats of political power. Highly skewed strategies of resolution favor the politically and financially powerful, and framing strategies are constructed to create division rather than community. We know this and are nonetheless astonished at the seeming incapacity of the American state to foster sustained moral obligation to and collective responsibility for the less fortunate who reside within its borders.

APPENDIX A

Chronologies

	France	United States
1982	July: Informal AIDS task force created within DGS.	July: CDC publishes account of three cases of pneumocystic pneumonia (PCP) among hemophiliacs, stating that "*although the cause of the severe immune dysfunction is unknown, the occurrence among the three hemophiliac cases suggests the possible transmission of an agent through blood products.*"
1982		July: Open meeting of PHS Committee on Opportunistic Infections in Patients with Hemophilia. Includes CDC, FDA, NIH, NHF, ARC, blood banking orgs., National Gay Task Force, NYCHD, NYC Inter-Hospital Study Group on AIDS. "*A possible mode of (AIDS) transmission is via blood products, in this case Factor VIII.*"
1983		January: CDC—Workgroup to Formulate Recommendations for Prevention of Acquired Immune Deficiency Syndrome (AIDS). No agreement. CDC: "*To bury our heads in the sand and say, 'Let's wait for more cases' is not an adequate public health measure.*"
1983	February: AIDS virus discovered by researchers at Institut Pasteur.	January: Joint statement of AABB, ARC, and CCBC. "*The possibility of blood borne transmission [of AIDS], still unproven, has been raised . . . there is no absolute evidence that AIDS is transmitted by blood or blood products. . . . Direct or indirect questions about a donor's sexual preference are inappropriate.*"
		March: FDA recommends "*educational programs*" informing persons "*at increased risk*" to refrain from blood or plasma donation.

	France	United States
1983	June: CNTS study reported to CCTS shows *"immune system anomalies"* among hemophiliacs, including those using only French blood.	May: NHF recommends hemophilia patients maintain use of blood product (Factor VIII) if recommended by their physicians.
1983	June: Board chair of CCTS tells AFH national meeting, *"hepatitis is more to be feared than AIDS."*	July: FDA internal memo: *"the benefit from life-threatening or disabling hemorrhage far exceeds the risk of acquiring AIDS."*
1983	June: Publication of DGS circular on donor selection	
1984		October: NHF: *"treaters . . . should strongly consider changing to heat-treated products."*
1985		April: Blood testing for HIV begins.
1985	May: "Confidential." CNTS meeting. *"All our lots are contaminated. . . . What position should the CNTS take with respect to products prepared with HIV+ plasma?"* Issues are financial. Decision bumped to government (*autorités de tutelles*).	
1985	July: Arrêté du 23 Juillet 1985. As of August 1, 1985, all blood donations from voluntary blood donors must be screened for HIV. Arrêté du 23 Juillet 1985. As of October 1, 1985, health insurance will no longer pay for non-heat-treated products.	December: California court finds plaintiff's lawsuit against Hyland Therapeutics based on strict liability is prohibited by California's blood shield law. (*Hyland Therapeutics v. Superior Ct.*, 220 Cal. Rptr. 590 (Cal. App. Ct. 1985).
1987	Militant hemophiliac group organized in Paris.	Publication of *And the Band Played On* by Randy Shilts.
1988	HIV + hemophiliacs launch lawsuits.	
1989	April: Publication in *Le Monde*: "The Scandal of Hemophiliacs."	September: Gaul exposé of blood business in *Philadelphia Inquirer*.
1990		July: First Dingell hearing on "Blood Supply Safety."
1990		August: Ryan White Care Act passed.
1991	May: Publication in *L'Événement du jeudi* of May 1985 internal CNTS memo on HIV contamination of blood products.	Militant hemophiliac groups organized in Boston and California.
1991	June: Resignation of Michel Garretta as head of CNTS.	

	France	United States
M1991	**September:** Publication of Lucas report: *Transfusion sanguine et sida en 1985 (Blood Transfusion and AIDS in 1985)*.	
1991	**December:** Senate creates Commission d'enquéte sur le système transfusionnel français en vue de son éventuelle réforme (Commission of Inquiry on the French Transfusion System with a View to Its Reform).	
1991	**December:** Law passed to compensate HIV-infected hemophiliacs, transfusees, part- ners, children, and heirs.	
1992	**June:** Publication of Senate Commission report: La crise du systeme transfusionnel français (*The Crisis of the French Transfusion System*)	**May:** Militant hemophiliacs call for con- gressional investigation of HIV/blood contamination.
1992	**June:** Opening in Paris of trial of blood and public health officials (Garretta, Allain, Roux, and Netter).	
1992	**October:** 3 of 4 officials found guilty of (1) "merchandising fraud" (Garretta and Allain) and (2) "non-assistance to persons in danger" (Roux). Garretta goes to prison.	
1993	**February:** Publication of Assemblée Nationale Commission report: **Rapport** de la commis- sion d'enquête (1) sur l'état des **connaissances scientifiques** et les **actions menées** à l'égard de la **transmission du sida** au cours des **dix dernières années** en France et à l'étranger *Inquiry on the State of Scientific Knowledge and Actions Taken on the Transmission of AIDS over the Past 10 Years in France and Other Countries.*	

	France	United States
1993	**December.** Law passed to reform blood system and created pharmaceutical drugs agency.	**April:** Letter to secretary of DHHS (Donna Shalala) from Senators Kennedy and Graham and Representative Goss requesting investigation of "*the issue of HIV transmission among hemophiliacs through contaminated blood products.*"
1993		**July:** Letter from Shalala to Goss referring matter to IOM.
1993		**September:** Militant hemophiliacs file class action suit against blood product manufacturers and NHF.
1995		**March:** On appeal, class is decertified and the matter returned to lower court.
1995		**July:** Publication of IOM report: *HIV and the Blood Supply: An Analysis of Crisis Decisionmaking.*
1995		**February:** Ricky Ray Act to compensate hemophiliacs is introduced in Congress.
1998		**November:** Ricky Ray Act signed into law.
1999	Cases against prime minister and health minister in 1985 dismissed.	
2002	All remaining toxic blood cases dismissed.	

APPENDIX B

Acronyms

AABB   American Association of Blood Banks
AAPHR American Association of Physicians for Human Rights
ABC   American Blood Commission
ABRA   American Blood Resources Association
ADP   Association de Défense des Polytransfusées
ADT   Association des Transfusées
AFH   Association Française des Hémophiles
AFLS   Agence Française de Lutte Contre le Sida
AHF   Anti-Hemophilia Factor
AN   Assemblée Nationale
ARC   American National Red Cross
ARSIDA Association de recherche sur le sida (French Working Group on AIDS)
BPAC   Blood Products Advisory Committee
CBER   Center for Biologics Evaluation and Research (formerly, Bureau of Biologics)
CCBC   Council of Community Blood Centers
CCNE   Comité consultative national d'éthique
CCTS   Commission Consultative de Transfusion Sanguine
CDC   (U.S.) Centers for Disease Control and Prevention
CNTS   Centre National de Transfusion Sanguine
COTT   Committee of Ten Thousand
CTS   Centre de Transfusion Sanguine
DDASS Direction Départementale des Affaires Sanitaires et Sociales
DGS   Direction Générale de la Santé
DRASS Direction Régionale des Affaires Sanitaires et Sociales
FDA   (U.S.) Food and Drug Administration
FFDSB Fédération Française des Donneurs de Sang Bénévoles
FNA   French National Archives
IGAS   Inspection Générale des Affaires Sociales
IOM   (U.S.) Institute of Medicine
JOR   *Journal Officiel de la République*
LNS   Laboratoire Nationale de la Santé
MMWR   (U.S.) *Morbidity and Mortality Weekly Report*
MOH   (French) Ministry of Health
NHF   National Hemophilia Foundation
PEER   HIV Peer Association

APPENDIX C
Original Sources

France

On-site or in person

French National Archives—Fontainebleau*
French National Archives—Pierrefitte-sur-Seine*
Librairie du Sénat
Bibliothèque Sciences Po
Bibliothèque St. Géneviève
Oral histories (10)

Electronic

Assemblée Nationale—http://www.assemblee-nationale.fr
Sénat—http://www.senat.fr
LexisNexis Academic (Columbia University Library)
Figaro microfiche collection (Columbia University Library)

Other

IGAS—document transmission by surface mail
Cour des comptes—document transmission by email

United States

On-site or in person

U.S. National Archives (Curran Archives)—Atlanta, GA
National Academy of Sciences (IOM blood committee archives)—Washington, D.C.
Columbia Center for Oral History (Resnik oral history archives)—New York City. Cited as Resnik Archives.
Harvard University Countway Library (Brandt archives)—Boston, MA
Oral histories (4)

Electronic

Emory Center for Digital Scholarship (CDC oral history archives—https://globalhealt hchronicles.org). Cited as CDC/Emory Archives.
ProQuest Historical Newspapers (Columbia University Library)

Other

San Francisco Public Library (Shilts Archives)—document transmission by surface mail. Cited as Shilts Archives.
*In the course of our research the relevant archives were moved from the Fountainebleau to the Pierrefitte site.

Bibliography

Abolafia, Mitchel Y. 2020. *Stewards of the Market: How the Federal Reserve Made Sense of the Financial Crisis*. Cambridge, MA: Harvard University Press.

Alam, Thomas. 2010. "Les mises en forme savante d'un mythe d'action publique: la sécurité sanitaire." *Genèses* 78:48–66.

Alam, Thomas, and Godard, Jérôme. 2007. "Réformes sectorielles et monstration de la modernité. Les usages des savoirs managériaux dans les politiques de l'emploi et de l'alimentation." *Politix* 79:77–100.

Alexander, Jeffrey C. 2010. *The Civil Sphere*. New York: Oxford University Press.

Alexander, Jeffrey C. 2018. "The Societalization of Social Problems: Church Pedophilia, Phone Hacking, and the Financial Crisis." *American Sociological Review* 83(6):1049–78.

Alexander, Jeffrey C. 2019. *What Makes a Social Crisis? The Societalization of Social Problems*. Cambridge: Polity Press.

Andrews, William G., and Hoffman, Stanley, eds. 1981. *The Fifth Republic at Twenty*. Albany: State University of New York Press.

Appadurai, Arjun. 1986. "Introduction: Commodities and the Politics of Value." Pp. 3–63 in *The Social Life of Things: Commodities in Cultural Perspective*, edited by Arjun Appadurai. Cambridge: Cambridge University Press.

Armstrong, Elizabeth A. 2002. *Forging Gay Identities: Organizing Sexuality in San Francisco, 1950–1994*. Chicago: University of Chicago Press.

Assemblée Nationale. 1993. *L'état des connaissances scientifiques et les actions menées à l'égard de la transmission du sida au cours des dix dernières années en France et à l'étranger*. Report # 3252. Paris: Assemblée Nationale. (Published in the *Journal Officiel* on February 5.)

Baldwin, Peter. 2005. *Disease and Democracy: The Industrialized World Faces AIDS*. Berkeley: University of California Press.

Balter, Michael. 1994. "French AIDS Scandal: Letters Provoke Unintended Response." *Science*, January 28.

Bayer, Ronald. 1997. "Review: HIV and the Blood Supply: An Analysis of Crisis Decisionmaking." *American Journal of Public Health* 87(3):474–76.

Bayer, Ronald. 1999. "Blood and AIDS in America: Science, Politics, and the Making of a Iatrogenic Catastrophe." Pp. 20–58 in *Blood Feuds: AIDS, Blood, and the Politics of Medical Disaster*, edited by Eric A. Feldman and Ronald Bayer. New York: Oxford University Press.

Bayer, Ronald, and David L. Kirp. 1992. "The United States: At the Center of the Storm." Pp. 7–48, *AIDS in the Industrialized Democracies: Passions, Politics, and Policies*, edited by David L. Kirp and Ronald Bayer. New Brunswick, NJ: Rutgers University Press.

Beaud, Olivier. 1999. *Le sang contaminé: essai critique sur la criminalisation de la responsabilité des gouvernants*. Paris: Presses Universitaires de France.

Beckert, Jens. 2010. "How Do Fields Change? The Interrelations of Institutions, Networks, and Cognition in the Dynamics of Markets." *Organization Studies* 31(05):605–27.

Bell, John, Sophie Boyron, and Simon Whittaker. 2008. *Principles of French Law*. 2nd ed. New York: Oxford University Press.

Benford, Robert D., and David A. Snow. 2000. "Framing Processes and Social Movements: An Overview and Assessment." *Annual Review of Sociology* 26:611–39.

Benamouzig, Daniel, and Julien Besançon. 2005. "Administrer un monde incertain: les nouvelles bureaucraties techniques. Le cas des agences sanitaires en France." *Sociologie du Travail* 47:301–322.

Bergeron, Henri. 2007. "Les transformations du colloque singulier médecin/patient: quelques perspectives sociologiques." Pp. 35–47 in *Les droits des malades et des usagers du système de santé, une législature plus tard*, edited by Didier Tabuteau. Paris: Presses de Sciences Po.

Bergeron, Henri. 2013. "Les mouvements sociaux sont-ils solubles dans le droit des patients." Pp. 89–102 in *La loi de 4 mars 2002 relative aux droits des malades: 10 ans après*, edited by Mireille Baccache, Anne Laude, and Didier Tabuteau. Brussels: Editions Bruylant.

Bergeron, Henri, Olivier Borraz, Patrick Castel, and François Dedieu. 2020. *Covid-19: une crise organisationnelle*. Paris: Sciences Po.

Bergeron, Henri, and Patrick Castel. 2014. Sociologie politique de la santé. Paris: Presses Universitaires de France.

Bergeron, Henri, H., and Constance A. Nathanson. 2012. "Construction of a Policy Arena: The Case of Public Health in France." *Journal of Health Politics, Policy and Law* 37(1):5–36.

Bergeron, Henri, and Constance A. Nathanson. 2014. "Faire une loi, pour faire la loi. La loi de santé publique d'août 2004." *Sciences Sociales et Santé* 32(4):5–32.

Berlivet, Luc. 2000. "Une santé à risques. L'action publique contre l'alcoolisme et le tabagisme en France (1954–1999)." PhD diss., Université de Rennes I.

Best, Rachel Kahn. 2019. *Common Enemies: Disease Campaigns in America*. New York: Oxford University Press.

Blin, Yves, and René Bestaux. 1971. "L'organisation et le fonctionnement de services et organismes de transfusion sanguine." Pp. 177–96 in *Comité central d'enquête sur le coût et le rendement des services publics*. Paris: Services du Premier Ministre.

Borraz, Olivier. 2008. *Les politiques du risque*. Paris: Presses de Sciences Po.

Borraz, Olivier, and Claude Gilbert. 2008. "Quand l'État prend des risques." Pp. 337–57 in *Politiques publiques. 1. La France dans la gouvernance européenne*, edited by Olivier Borraz and Virginie Guiraudon. Paris: Presses de Sciences Po.

Borsa, Alexander, and Joseph Dov Bruch. 2022. "Prevalence and Performance of Private Equity-Affiliated Fertility Practices in the United States." *Fertility and Sterility* 117(1):124–30.

Bourdieu, Pierre. 2014. *On the State*. Translated by David Fernbach. Cambridge: Polity Press.

Broqua, Christophe. 2020. *Action=Vie. A History of AIDS Activism and Gay Politics in France*. Translated from the French by Jean-Yves Bart and Kel Pero. Philadelphia: Temple University Press.

Bruch, Joseph D., Alexander Borsa, Zirui Song, and Sarah S. Richardson. 2020. "Expansion of Private Equity Involvement in Women's Health Care." *JAMA Internal Medicine* 180(11):1542–45.

Burawoy, Michael. 1998. "The Extended Case Method." *Sociological Theory* 16(1):4–33.

Buton, François. 2005. "Sida et politique: saisir les formes de la lutte." *Revue Française de Science Politique* 55(5–6):787–810.

Callon, Michel, Piérre Lascoumes, and Yannick Barthe. 2001. *Agir dans un monde incertain: Essai sur la démocratie technique.* Paris: Le Seuil.

Camus, Albert. 1948. *The Plague.* Vintage International. New York: Alfred A. Knopf.

Carpenter, Daniel. 2010. *Reputation and Power: Organizational Image and Pharmaceutical Regulation at the FDA.* Princeton: Princeton University Press.

Carricaburu, Danièle. 2000. *L'hémophile au risque de la médecine: de la maladie individuelle à la contamination collective par le virus du Sida.* Paris: Anthropos.

Casassus, Barbara. 2003. "French Supreme Court Ends Tainted Blood Saga." *Science* 300 (5628), June 27:2019.

Casteret, Anne-Marie. 1992. *L'affaire du sang.* Paris: Éditions La Découverte.

Casteret, Anne-Marie. 1991. "Le rapport qui accuse le Centre National de Transfusion Sanguine." *L'Évènement du Jeudi.* April 25, 1991.

Centers for Disease Control. 1982. "Pneumocystis Carnii Pneumonia among Persons with Hemophilia A." *Morbidity and Mortality Weekly Report* 31(27):365–67.

Centers for Disease Control. 1983. "Prevention of Acquired Immune Deficiency Syndrome: Report of Inter-Agency Recommendations." *Morbidity and Mortality Weekly Report* 32(8):101–3.

Cerny, Philip G., and Martin A. Schain, eds. 1980. *French Politics and Public Policy.* New York: St. Martin's Press.

Chambré, Susan M. 2006. *Fighting for Our Lives: New York's AIDS Community and the Politics of Disease.* New Brunswick, NJ: Rutgers University Press.

Champagne, Patrick, and Dominique Marchetti. 1994. "L'information médicale sous contrainte a propos du 'scandale du sang contaminé.'" *Actes de La Recherche En Sciences Sociales* 101(1):40–62.

Chapoutot, Johann. 2014. *La loi du sang: Penser et agir en Nazi.* Paris: Editions Gallimard.

Chauveau, Sophie. 2004. "Genèse de la 'sécurité sanitaire': Les produits pharmaceutiques en France aux XIXe et XXe siècles." *Revue d'Histoire Moderne et Contemporaine* 52(2):88–117.

Chauveau, Sophie. 2007. "Du don au marché: politiques du sang en France années 1940–années 2000." Habilitation à Diriger des Recherches. Paris, École des Hautes Études en Sciences Sociales.

Chauveau, Sophie. 2011. *L'affaire du sang contaminé (1983–2003).* Paris: Les Belles Lettres.

Clemens, Elizabeth S., and James M Cook. 1999. "Politics and Institutionalism: Explaining Durability and Change." *Annual Review of Sociology* 25:441–66.

Cohen, Stanley. 2001. *States of Denial: Knowing About Atrocities and Suffering.* Cambridge: Polity Press.

Cohen-Tanugi, Laurent. 1996. "The Law Without the State." Pp. 269–73 in *European Legal Cultures,* edited by Volkmar Gessner, Armin Hoeland, and Csaba Varga. Aldershot, UK: Dartmouth.

Colgrove, James. 2006. *State of Immunity: The Politics of Vaccination in Twentieth-Century America.* Berkeley: University of California Press.

Congressional Record. 101st Congress (1989–90)—Thomas (Library of Congress).

Council of Europe. 1983. Ministers' Committee. June 23.

Cour des comptes. 2017. "L'indemnisation amiable des victimes d'accidents médicaux: une mise en œuvre dévoyée, une remise en ordre impérative." Paris: Cour des Comptes.

Crozier, Michel. 2017. *The Bureaucratic Phenomenon*. New York: Routledge. (Published originally in 1964 as *Phénomène bureaucratique*.)

Cunningham v. MacNeal Memorial Hospital. 1970. 266 N.E.2d 897, 904 (Illinois).

Curran, James W. 1987. Statement of James W. Curran, M.D., Director, AIDS Program, Center for Infectious Diseases, Centers for Disease Control, Public Health Service, U.S. Department of Health and Human Services. Committee on Veterans' Affairs, U.S. Senate, June 24, 1987.

Cusset, François. 2006. *La décennie: Le grand cauchemar des années 1980*. Paris: La Découverte.

Cutter Laboratories. 1983. "National Hemophilia Foundation/Industry Strategy Meeting on AIDS." New York City, January 14.

Davidson, Michael. 2008. "Strange Blood: Hemophobia and the Unexplored Boundaries of Queer Nation." Pp. 35–57 in *Concerto for the Left Hand: Disability and the Defamiliar Body*. Ann Arbor: University of Michigan Press.

DePrince, Elaine. 1997. *Cry Bloody Murder: A Tale of Tainted Blood*. New York: Random House.

"Disease Stirs Fear on Blood Supply." 1983. *New York Times*, January 6, 1983:B17.

Donovan, Mark C. 1996. "The Politics of Deservedness: The Ryan White Act and the Social Constructions of People with AIDS." Pp 68–87 in *AIDS: The Politics and Policy of Disease*, edited by Stella Theodoulou. Upper Saddle River, NJ: Prentice Hall.

Donovan, Mark C. 2001. *Taking Aim: Target Populations and the War on AIDS and Drugs*. Washington, D.C.: Georgetown University Press.

Dorney, Linda M. 1994. "Culpable Conduct with Impunity: The Blood Industry and the FDA'S Responsibility for the Spread of AIDS Through Blood Products." *Journal of Pharmacy & Law* 3:129–80.

Douglas, Mary. 1992. *Risk and Blame: Essays in Cultural Theory*. London: Routledge.

Drake, Donald C. 1983. "The Disease Detectives Puzzle over Methods of Control." *Philadelphia Inquirer*, January 9, 1983.

Duchesne, Sophie. 1997. *Citoyenneté à la Française*. Paris: Presses de Sciences Po.

Dulac, Fabienne. 1992. "De refus de la maladie a une prise en charge exigeante: Le role des associations issues des milieux homosexuels." Pp. 61–73 in *Sida et politique: les premiers affrontements (1981–1987)*, edited by Pierre Favre. Paris: Editions L'Harmattan.

Eckert, Ross D. 1992. "The AIDS Blood-Transfusion Cases: A Legal and Economic Analysis of Liability." *San Diego Law Review* 29:203–98.

Epstein, Steven. 1996. *Impure Science: AIDS, Activism, and the Politics of Knowledge*. Berkeley: University of California Press.

Erikson, Kai. 1976. *Everything in Its Path: Destruction of Community in the Buffalo Creek Flood*. New York: Simon and Schuster.

Evin, Claude. 1989. "Préface." Pp. 9–13 in *Rapport sur le SIDA: 23 août–3 octobre 1988*, edited by Claude Got. Paris: Flammarion.

Eyal, Gil. 2019. *The Crisis of Expertise*. Cambridge: Polity Press.

Fairchild, Amy, Constance A. Nathanson, and Cullen Conway. 2021. "Fear and Panic at the Borders: Outbreak Anxieties in the United States from the Colonies to COVID-19." Pp. 199–224 in *Medicalising Borders: Selection, Containment and Quarantine Since 1800*, edited by Sevasti Trubeta, Christian Promitzer, and Paul Weindling. Manchester: Manchester University Press.

Feldman, Eric A. 2000. "Blood Justice: Courts, Conflict, and Compensation in Japan, France, and the United States." *Law & Society Review* 34(3):651–701.

Feldman, Eric A., and Ronald Bayer. 1999. *Blood Feuds: AIDS, Blood, and the Politics of Medical Disaster*. New York: Oxford University Press.

Figaro. 1991. "La gendarmerie réclame des inculpations." June 5, 1991:3.

Fillion, Emmanuelle. 2009. *À L 'épreuve du sang contaminé: pour une sociologie des affaires médicales*. Paris: École des Hautes Études en Sciences Sociales.

Fine, Gary Alan. 2019. "Moral Cultures, Reputation Work, and the Politics of Scandal." *Annual Review of Sociology* 45:247–64.

Fligstein, Neil, and Doug McAdam. 2012. *A Theory of Fields*. Oxford: Oxford University Press.

Food and Drug Administration. Bureau of Biologics. Blood Products Advisory Committee. 1983. "Closed Session VIII: General Discussion." February 7, 1983. (BPAC)

Fourcade, Marion. 2011. "Cents and Sensibility: Economic Valuation and the Nature of 'Nature.'" *American Journal of Sociology* 116(6):1721–77.

Franklin, Marc A. 1972. "Tort Liability for Hepatitis: An Analysis and a Proposal." *Stanford Law Review* 24(3):439–80.

Freidson, Eliot. 1970. *Professional Dominance: The Social Structure of Medical Care*. New York: Atherton Press.

Gabriel, Yiannis. 2004. "Narratives, Stories, and Texts." Pp. 61–77 in *The Sage Handbook of Organizational Discourse*, edited by David Grant, Cynthia Hardy, Cliff Oswick, and Linda Putnam. London: SAGE.

Gamson, William A. 1992. "The Social Psychology of Collective Action." Pp. 53–76 in *Frontiers in Social Movement Theory*, edited by Aldon D. Morris and Carol McClurg Mueller. New Haven: Yale University Press.

Gaul, Gilbert M. 1989a. "Fear of AIDS Spurs Change." *Philadelphia Inquirer*, September 26, 1989:1.

Gaul, Gilbert M. 1989b. "How Blood, the 'Gift of Life,' Became a Billion Dollar Business." *Philadelphia Inquirer*, September 24,1989:1.

Gaul, Gilbert M. 1989c. "Red Cross: From Disaster Relief to Blood." *Philadelphia Inquirer*, September 27, 1989:1.

Gaul, Gilbert M. 1989d. "The Loose Way the FDA Regulates the Blood Industry." *Philadelphia Inquirer*, September 25, 1989:1.

Gaul, Gilbert M. 1989e. "America: The OPEC of the Global Plasma Industry." *Philadelphia Inquirer*, September 28, 1989:1.

Girard, Jean-François. 1998. *Quand la santé déviant publique*. Paris: Hachette Littérature.

Glied, Sherry. 1996. "Markets Matter: U.S. Responses to the HIV-Infected Blood Tragedy." *Virginia Law Review* 82(8):1493–509.

Goldman, Meyer L. 1964. "Is Human Blood a Commodity?" *Transfusion* 4(3):207–8.

Got, Claude. 1989. *Rapport sur le SIDA: 23 Août–3 Octobre 1988*. Paris: Flammarion.

Greilsamer, Laurent. 1992. *Le procès du sang contaminé*. Paris: Le Monde Editions.

Grémy, François. 2004. *On a encore oublié la santé*. Paris: Éditions Frison-Roche.

Gusfield, Joseph R. 1981. *The Culture of Public Problems: Drinking-Driving and the Symbolic Order*. Chicago: University of Chicago Press.

Haas, Michael. 1992. *Polity and Society: Philosophical Underpinnings of Social Science Paradigms*. New York: Praeger.

Haines, Herbert H. 1984. "Black Radicalization and the Funding of Civil Rights: 1957–70." *Social Problems* 321(October):31–43.

Healy, Kieran. 2006. *Last Best Gifts: Altruism and the Market for Human Blood and Organs*. Chicago: University of Chicago Press.

Hermitte, Marie-Angèle. 1996. *Le sang et le droit: Essai sur la transfusion sanguine.* Paris: Seuil.

Herzlich, Claudine, and Janine Pierret. 1988. "Une maladie dans l'espace public. Le SIDA dans six quotidiens Français." *Annales. Economies, Sociétes, Civilisations* 43(5):1109–34.

Hilgartner, Stephen. 2000. *Science on Stage: Expert Advice as Public Drama.* Stanford, CA: Stanford University Press.

Hilgartner, Stephen, and Charles L Bosk. 1988. "The Rise and Fall of Social Problems: A Public Arenas Model." *American Journal of Sociology* 94(1):53–78.

Hilts, Philip J. 2003. *Protecting America's Health: The FDA, Business, and One Hundred Years of Regulation.* Chapel Hill: University of North Carolina Press.

Hoffmann, Stanley. 1980. "Preface: France's Condition, 1980." Pp. vi–xiii in *French Politics and Public Policy*, edited by Philip G. Cerny and Martin A. Schain. New York: St. Martin's Press.

"Human Rights—AIDS." 1983. *Colorado Gay and Lesbian News*, May 1983.

In the Matter of Community Blood Bank of the Kansas City Area Inc., et al. 1966. Docket 8519. Complaint, July 5, 1962, Decision, Sept. 28, 1966. (70 FTC).

In the Matter of Rhone-Poulenc Rorer Incorporated, et al. 1995. U.S. Court of Appeals, 7th Cir., March 16, 1995.

Institute of Medicine. 1994. Committee to Study HIV Transmission Through Blood Products, Public Meeting, September 12. U.S. Department of Commerce, National Technical Information Service.

Institute of Medicine. 1995. *HIV and the Blood Supply: An Analysis of Crisis Decisionmaking.* Washington, D.C: National Academy Press.

Institute of Medicine, National Academy of Sciences, Division of Health Promotion and Disease Prevention. 1994. Committee to Study HIV Transmission Through Blood Products Public Meeting. PB95142345. Washington, D.C: National Academy of Sciences.

Jaffee, Daniel, and Howard, Philip H. 2009. "Corporate Cooptation of Organic and Fair Trade Standards." *Agriculture and Human Values* 17(3):387–99.

Jankowski, Paul. 2008. *Shades of Indignation: Political Scandals in France, Past and Present.* New York: Berghahn Books.

Jasanoff, Sheila. 1990. *The Fifth Branch: Science Advisors as Policymakers.* Cambridge, MA: Harvard University Press.

Jasanoff, Sheila. 1995. *Science at the Bar: Law, Science, and Technology in America.* Cambridge, MA: Harvard University Press.

Jasanoff, Sheila. 2005. *Designs on Nature: Science and Democracy in Europe and the United States.* Princeton: Princeton University Press.

Kaufman, Marc. 2001. "Seeking Compassionate Compensation; Transfusion-Acquired AIDS Patients Want Same Right as Hemophiliacs." *Washington Post*, January 2, 2001:3.

Kennedy, Louanne. 1978. "Community Blood Banking in the United States from 1937–1975: Organizational Formation, Transformation, and Reform in a Climate of Competing Ideologies." PhD diss., New York University.

Keshavjeea, Salmaan, Sherri Weiserb, and Arthur Kleinman. 2001. "Medicine Betrayed: Hemophilia Patients and HIV in the US." *Social Science & Medicine* 53:1081–94.

Kessler, David. 2001. *A Question of Intent.* New York: BBS Publications.

Kitschelt, Herbert P. 1986. "Political Opportunity Structures and Political Protest: Anti-Nuclear Movements in Four Democracies." *British Journal of Political Science* 16(1):57–85.

Klein, Andrew. 1995. "Compensate AIDS Stricken Hemophiliacs." *Philadelphia Inquirer*, August 5, 1995:9 (Editorial).

Klinenberg, Eric. 2002. *Heat Wave: A Social Autopsy of Disaster in Chicago*. Chicago: University of Chicago Press.

Korner, Barbara L., Philip S. Rosenberg, Louis M. Aledort, et al. 1994. "HIV-1 Infection Incidence Among Persons with Hemophilia in the United States and Western Europe, 1978–1990." *Journal of Acquired Immune Deficiency Syndrome* 7:279–86.

Kouchner, Bernard. 1993. "Préface." Pp. 9–11 in *Le problème Français des accidents thérapeutiques: enjeux et solutions*, François Ewald. Paris: Ministère de la santé et de l'action humanitaire.

Kramer, Jane. 1993. "Bad Blood." *New Yorker*, October 11, 1993:74–95.

Kuhn, Dana. 1995. "The Trail of AIDS in the Hemophilia Community." 3rd ed. Published by the Committee of Ten Thousand.

Lachenal, Guillaume, and Gaetan Thomas. 2020. "Epidemics Have Lost the Plot." *Bulletin of the History of Medicine* 94(4):670–89.

Lamont, Michèle. 1992. *Money, Morals, and Manners: The Culture of the French and the American Upper-Middle Class*. Chicago: University of Chicago Press.

Lamont, Michèle. 2000. *The Dignity of Working Men: Morality and the Boundaries of Race, Class, and Immigration*. New York: Russell Sage Foundation.

Lamont, Michèle, and Thévenot, Laurent. 2000. *Rethinking Comparative Cultural Sociology: Repertoires of Evaluation in France and the United States*. Cambridge: Cambridge University Press.

Lascoumes, Pierre. 1996. "La précaution comme anticipation des risques résiduels et hybridation de la responsabilité." *L'Année Sociologique* 46(2):359–82.

Lederer, Susan. 2008. *Flesh and Blood: Organ Transplantation and Blood Transfusion in 20th Century America*. New York: Oxford University Press.

Leibowitch, Jacques. 1984. *Un virus étrange venu d'ailleurs*. Paris: Grasset.

Lewis, Anthony. 1995. "Reform or Wreck?" *New York Times*, January 27, 1995.

Lofland, John. 1996. *Social Movement Organizations*. New York: Aldine de Gruyter.

Lucas, Michel. 1991. *Transfusion sanguine et Sida en 1985: chronologie des faits et des décisions pour ce qui concerne les hémophiles*. Paris: Inspection Générale des Affaires Sociales.

Marchetti, Dominique. 2010. *Quand la santé devient médiatique: les logiques de production de l'information dans la presse*. Grenoble: Presses Universitaires de Grenoble.

Marmor, Theodore R., Patricia A. Dillon, and Stephen Scher. 1999. "Conclusion: The Comparative Politics of Contaminated Blood: From Hesitancy to Scandal." Pp. 349–66 in *Blood Feuds: AIDS, Blood, and the Politics of Medical Disaster*, edited by Eric. A. Feldman and Ronald Bayer. New York: Oxford University Press.

Mathiot, Pierre. 1992. "Le Sida dans la stratégie et la rhétorique du Front National." Pp. 189–201 in *Sida et politique: les premiers affrontements (1981–1987)*, edited by Pierre Favre. Paris: Editions L'Harmattan.

McAdam, Doug, and W. Richard Scott. 2005. "Organizations and Movements." Pp. 4–40 in *Social Movements and Organization Theory*, edited by Gerald Davis et al. New York: Columbia University Press.

Morelle, Aquilino. 1996. *La défaite de la santé publique*. Paris: Flammarion.

Morris, Aldon D. 1993. "Birmingham Confrontation Reconsidered: An Analysis of the Dynamics and Tactics of Mobilization." *American Sociological Review* 58(5):621–36.

Mulcahy, Andrew W. et al. 2016. *Toward a Sustainable Blood Supply in the United States*. Santa Monica, CA: Rand Corporation.

Muller, Jean-Yves. 2004. "Jean-Pierre Soulier (1915–2003). Une évocation de l'œuvre scientifique et médicale de Jean-Pierre Soulier." *Transfusion Clinique et Biologique* 11:57–64.

Murard, Lion, and Patrick Zylberman. 1996. *L'hygiène dans la république*. Paris: Fayard.

Nathanson, Constance A. 2007. *Disease Prevention as Social Change: The State, Society, and Public Health in the United States, France, Great Britain, and Canada*. New York: Russell Sage Foundation.

Nathanson, Constance A., and Henri Bergeron. 2017. "Crisis and Change: The Making of a French FDA." *The Milbank Quarterly* 95(3):634–75.

National Research Council. 1970. *Evaluation of the Utilization of Human Blood Resources in the United States (1970)*. Washington, D.C: National Academies Press.

Nau, Jean-Yves. 1989. "Sida: le scandale des hémophiles." *Le Monde*, April 28, 1989:19.

Nau, Jean-Yves. 1990. "Sida: le don du mal Le risque du sida après transfusion sanguine ne semble pas décroitre en France. Une nouvelle association de défense des victimes vient de se créer." *Le Monde*, February 28, 1990.

Nau, Jean-Yves. 1992. "Contamination: le sang des prisons. La forte proportion de personnes infectées en France par le virus du sida à la suite d'une transfusion s'explique en partie par les collectes effectuées en milieu pénitentiaire." *Le Monde*, April 11, 1992.

Nau, Jean-Yves, and Franck Nouchi. 1991a. "Un entretien avec M. Bruno Durieux." *Le Monde*, June 7, 1991.

Nau, Jean-Yves, and Franck Nouchi. 1991b. "L'affaire des dons de sang contaminé. Sida et transfusion: les étapes d'une catastrophe." *Le Monde*, June 18, 1991.

Nau, Jean-Yves, and Franck Nouchi. 1991c. "Un système archaïque." *Le Monde*, October 22, 1991.

Nau, Jean-Yves, and Franck Nouchi. 1991d. " La santé défaillante." *Le Monde*, November 5, 1991.

Nau, Jean-Yves, and Franck Nouchi. 1992. "Contamination: le sang des prisons Querelles de spécialistes, lenteurs administratives, volonté de ne pas aggraver les tensions en milieu carcéral: ce n'est qu'après l'été 1985 que les collectes " à risques " prirent fin." *Le Monde*, April 15, 1992.

Neustadt, Richard A., and Harvey Fineberg. 1978. *The Swine Flu Affair: Decision-Making on a Slippery Disease*. Washington, D.C: U.S. Department of Health, Education, and Welfare.

Nohrstedt, Daniel, and Christopher M. Weible. 2010. "The Logic of Policy Change After Crisis: Proximity and Subsystem Interaction." *Risk, Hazards & Crisis in Public Policy* 1(2):1–32.

Nothias, Jean-Luc. 1991a. "Comment le silence des contaminés était 'acheté." *Figaro*, June 10, 1991.

Nothias, Jean-Luc. 1991b. "Le président de l'Association de défense des transfusées envisage d'appeler au boycottage des dons de sang." *Figaro*, July 16, 1991:8.

Nouchi, Franck. 1991a. "Publié par *L'Événement du jeudi*. Un rapport met en cause le Centre national de transfusion sanguine." *Le Monde*, April 26, 1991.

Nouchi, Franck. 1991b. "L'affaire du sang contaminé. Un entretien avec le docteur Bahman Habibi." *Le Monde*, November 2, 1991.

Nouchi, Franck, and Jean-Yves Nau. 1991a. "Annoncée par M. Bruno Durieux la réforme du système de transfusion sanguine visera à garantir 'La plus Grande Sécurité Possible.'" *Le Monde*, November 5, 1991.

Nouchi, Franck, and Jean-Yves Nau. 1991b. "Selon le rapport de l'inspection Générale des Affaires Sociales des erreurs collectives sont en partie à l'origine de la contamination d'hémophiles par le virus du Sida." *Le Monde*, September 11, 1991.

Novak, William J. 2008. "The Myth of the 'Weak' American State." *American Historical Review* 113(3):752–72.

Parthasarathy, Shobita. 2017. *Patent Politics: Life Forms, Markets and the Public Interest in the United States and Europe.* Chicago: University of Chicago Press.

Péchu, Cécile. 1992. "Tenir le politique à l'écart: jeux et enjeux du travail médical." Pp. 41–58 in *Sida et politique: Les premiers affrontements (1981–1987)*, edited by Pierre Favre. Paris: Editions L'Harmattan.

Perlmutter v. Beth David Hospital. 1954. Court of Appeals of New York. 308 N.Y. 100, 123 N.E.2d 792.

Pinell, Patrice. 2002. *Une épidémie politique: la lutte contre le SIDA en France, 1981–1996.* Paris: Presses Universitaires de France.

Poumadère, Marc, and Claire Mays. 2003. "The Dynamics of Risk Amplification and Attenuation in Context: A French Case Study." Pp. 209–242 in *The Social Amplification of Risk*, edited by Nick Pidgeon, Roger E. Kasperson, and Paul Slovic. Cambridge: Cambridge University Press.

Prasad, Monica. 2012. *The Land of Too Much: American Abundance and the Paradox of Poverty.* Cambridge, MA: Harvard University Press.

Prearo, Massimo. 2014. *Le moment politique de l'homosexualité. Mouvements, identités et communautés en France.* Lyon: Presses Universitaires de Lyon.

Pryma, Jane. 2022. "Technologies of Expertise: Opioids and Pain Management's Credibility Crisis." *American Sociological Review* 87(1):1–33.

Quintana v. United Blood Services. 1991. Court of Appeals of Colo., Division 2, 811 P.2d 424.

Rabinow, Paul. 1999. *French DNA: Trouble in Purgatory.* Chicago: University of Chicago Press.

Ragin, Charles C., and Howard S. Becker. 1992. *What Is a Case? Exploring the Foundations of Social Inquiry.* Cambridge: Cambridge University Press.

Resnik, Susan. 1999. *Blood Saga: Hemophilia, AIDS, and the Survival of a Community.* Berkeley: University of California Press.

Richert, Lucas. 2014. *Conservatism, Consumer Choice, and the Food and Drug Administration During the Reagan Era: A Prescription for Scandal.* Lanham, MD: Lexington Books.

Riedmattan, Louis Armand. 1992. *L'affaire du sang contaminé.* Monaco: Editions du Rocher.

Rock, Andrea. 1986. "Inside the Billion Dollar Business of Blood." *Money*, March, 153–72.

Rosenberg, Charles. 1989. "What Is an Epidemic? AIDS in Historical Perspective." *Daedalus* (2):1–17.

Roux, Jacques. 1995. *Sang contaminé: priorités de l'État et décisions politiques.* Montpellier, France: Éditions Espace.

Rozenbaum, Willy, Didier Seux, and Annie Kouchner. 1984. *Sida, réalités et fantasmes.* Paris: POL.

Sahlins, Marshall. 1985. *Islands of History.* Chicago: University of Chicago Press.

Saul, Jessie E. 2004. "The Tainted Gift: A Comparative Study of the Culture and Politics of the Contamination of the Blood Supply with the AIDS Virus in France and the United States." PhD diss., Cornell University, Ithaca, NY.

Schmidt, Paul J. 1977. "National Blood Policy, 1977: A Study in the Politics of Health." *Progress in Hematology* 10:151–72.

Sénat (France) 1991a. "Débats Parlementaires." *Journal Officiel de la République Française*, November 17.

Sénat (France) 1991b. "Débats Parlementaires." *Journal Officiel de la République Française*, December 16.

Sénat (France). 1991c. "Débats Parlementaires." *Journal Officiel de la République Française*, December 17. (Statement of Jean-Louis Bianco.)

Sénat (France). 1992. *Rapport de La Commission d'enquête Sur Le Système Transfusionnel Français*. Report # 406. Paris. (Published in the *Journal Officiel* on June 12, 1992.)

Seo, Myeong-Gu, and Douglas Creed. 2002. "Institutional Contradictions, Praxis, and Institutional Change: A Dialectical Perspective." *Academy of Management Review* 27(2):222–47.

Setbon, Michel. 1993. *Pouvoirs contre Sida: de la transfusion sanguine au dépistage: décisions et pratiques en France, Grande-Bretagne et Suède*. Paris: Seuil.

Sewell, William H., Jr. 1992. "A Theory of Structure: Duality, Agency, and Transformation." *American Journal of Sociology* 98(1):1–29.

Sewell, William H., Jr. 1996. "Historical Events as Transformations of Structures: Inventing Revolution at the Bastille." *Theory and Society* 25(6):841–81.

Sewell, William H., Jr. 2005. *Logics of History: Social Theory and Social Transformation*. Chicago: University of Chicago Press.

Seytre, Bernard. 1993. *Sida: les secrets d'une polémique, intérêts financiers et médias*. Paris: Presses Universitaires de France.

Sharp, Lesley A. 2000. "The Commodification of the Body and Its Parts." *Annual Review of Anthropology* 29:287–328.

Shaw, Donna. 1998. "Hemophiliacs with HIV Get a Boost." *Philadelphia Inquirer*, May 20, 1998:6.

Shilts, Randy. 1987. *And the Band Played On: People, Politics, and the AIDS Epidemic*. New York: Penguin Books.

Siplon, Patricia D. 2002. *AIDS and the Policy Struggle in the United States*. Washington, D.C.: Georgetown University Press.

Snow, David A., E. Burke Rochford, Steven K. Worden, and Robert D. Benford. 1986. "Frame Alignment Processes, Micromobilization, and Movement Participation." *American Sociological Review* 51(August):464–81.

Soulier, Jean-Pierre. 1992. *Sida et transfusion sanguine. Le droit à la vérité*. Paris: Editions Frison-Roche.

Sourdille, Jacques, and Claude Huriet. 1992. *La crise du système transfusionnel Français*. Paris: Éditions Economica.

Starr, Douglas H. (1998) 2002. *Blood: An Epic History of Medicine and Commerce*. New York: Harper Collins.

Starr, Paul. 1982. *The Social Transformation of American Medicine*. New York: Basic Books.

Steffen, Monika. 1999. "The Nation's Blood: Medicine, Justice, and the State in France." Pp. 95–126 in *Blood Feuds; AIDS, Blood, and the Politics of Medical Disaster*, edited by Feldman, Eric A. and Ronald Bayer. New York: Oxford University Press.

Stone, Deborah A. 1988. *Policy Paradox and Political Reason*. New York: Harper Collins.

Stone, Deborah A. 1989. "Causal Stories and the Formation of Policy Agendas." *Political Science Quarterly* 104(2):281–300.

Strazzulla, Jérôme. 1991a. "Transfusion et sida: de la dérive au scandale." *Figaro*, May 30, 1991.

Strazzulla, Jérôme. 1991b. "Sang et Sida: Durieux condamne la polémique." *Figaro*, June 3, 1991.

Strazzulla, Jérôme. 1991c. "Bruno Durieux change de ton." *Figaro*, June 5, 1991.

Strazzulla, Jérôme. 1993. *Le Sida, 1981–1985.* Paris: La Documentation Française.

Suleiman, Ezra N. 1974. *Politics, Power, and Bureaucracy in France: The Administrative Elite*. Princeton: Princeton University Press.

Swidler, Ann. 1986. "Culture in Action: Symbols and Strategies." *American Sociological Review* 51(2):273–86.

Tabuteau, Didier. 2006. *Les contes de Ségur: Les coulisses de la politique de santé.* Paris: Ophrys.

Tabuteau, Didier. 2007. "La sécurité sanitaire, réforme institutionnelle ou résurgence des politiques de santé publique." *Sève* 3(16):87–103.

Tabuteau, Didier, and Aquilino Morelle. 2017. *La santé publique*. Paris: Presses Universitaires de France.

Tarrow, Sidney. 1998. *Power in Movement: Social Movements and Contentious Politics*. 2nd ed. Cambridge: Cambridge University Press.

Thornton, Patricia H., Ocasio, William, and Lounsbury, Michael. 2012. *The Institutional Logics Perspective: A New Approach to Culture, Structure, and Process*. Oxford: Oxford University Press.

Tilly, Charles. 1986. *The Contentious French*. Cambridge: Harvard University Press.

Tilly, Charles, Louise Tilly, and Richard Tilly. 1975. *The Rebellious Century 1830–1930*. Cambridge, MA: Harvard University Press.

Titmuss, Richard M. (1970) 1997. *The Gift Relationship: From Human Blood to Social Policy*. Expanded and updated edition. New York: New Press.

Trebilcock, Michael, Robert Howse, and Ron Daniels. 1996. "Do Institutions Matter? A Comparative Pathology of the HIV-Infected Blood Tragedy." *Virginia Law Review* 82(8):1407–92.

Treichler, Paula A. 1987. "AIDS, Homophobia, and Biomedical Discourse: An Epidemic of Signification." *AIDS: Cultural Analysis/Cultural Activism* 43:31–70.

U.S. House of Representatives, Committee on Energy and Commerce, Subcommittee on Oversight and Investigations. 1990. *Blood Supply Safety*. Washington, D.C.: U.S. Government Printing Office, July 13, 1990. ("Dingell hearings").

U.S. House of Representatives, Committee on Energy and Commerce, Subcommittee on Oversight and Investigations. 1993. *Blood Supply Safety*. Washington, D.C.: U.S. Government Printing Office, July 28, 1993. ("Dingell hearings").

U.S. House of Representatives, Committee on Government Reform and Oversight, Subcommittee on Human Resources and Intergovernmental Relations. 1995. *Protecting the Nation's Blood Supply from Infectious Agents: New Standards to Meet New Threats*. Washington, D.C: Government Printing Office, October 12 and November 2, 1995.

U.S. House of Representatives, Committee on Energy and Commerce. 1994. *Report on the Activity of the Committee on Energy and Commerce for the 103d Congress, 1st Session*. 103–417. Washington, D.C: Government Printing Office.

U.S. House of Representatives, Committee on the Judiciary, Subcommittee on Immigration and Claims. 1996. *Ricky Ray Hemophilia Relief Fund Act of 1995*. Washington, D.C: Government Printing Office, September 19, 1996.

U.S. Senate, Subcommittee on Antitrust and Monopoly, Committee on the Judiciary. 1964. *Blood Banks and Antitrust Laws*. Washington, D.C.: Government Printing Office, August 1964.

U.S. Senate, Committee on Veteran's Affairs. 1987. Statement of James W. Curran.

U.S. Senate, Committee on Labor and Human Resources. 1997. *HIV/AIDS: Recent Developments and Future Opportunities*. Washington, D.C: Government Printing Office, October 30, 1997.

Vaughan, Diane. 1996. *The Challenger Launch Decision: Risky Technology, Culture, and Deviance at NASA*. Chicago: University of Chicago Press.

Vaughan, Diane. 2006. "The Social Shaping of Commission Reports." *Sociological Forum* 21(2):291–306.

Vogel, David. 2012. *The Politics of Precaution: Regulating Health, Safety, and Environmental Risks in Europe and the United States*. Princeton: Princeton University Press.

Weick, Karl E. 1993. "The Collapse of Sensemaking in Organizations: The Mann Gulch Disaster." *Administrative Science Quarterly* 38(4):628–52.

Weick, Karl E. 1995. *Sensemaking in Organizations*. Thousand Oaks, CA: SAGE.

Weir, Margaret, and Theda Skocpol. 1985. "State Structures and the Possibilities for 'Keynesian' Responses to the Great Depression in Sweden, Britain, and the United States." Pp. 107–68 in *Bringing the State Back In*, edited by Peter B. Evans, Dietrich Rueschemeyer, and Theda Skocpol. New York: Cambridge University Press.

Zelizer, Viviana A. 1988. "Beyond the Polemics on the Market: Establishing a Theoretical and Empirical Agenda." *Sociological Forum* 3(4):614–34.

Index

For the benefit of digital users, indexed terms that span two pages (e.g., 52–53) may, on occasion, appear on only one of those pages.

Tables and figures are indicated by *t* and *f* following the page number

direct consumer opposition, absence
of, 32–33
Illinois State Medical Society lobbying,
31–32
blood supply
FDA responsibility for regulation of,
14–15
government control of, 3n.6
U.S., internal competition for, 35
"Blood Supply Safety" congressional
hearings, Dingell and, 96–100,
99n.36, 101n.37, 174n.11
"Blood Transfusion and AIDS in 1985,"
("Lucas report"), 91
Blood Transfusion Commission. See
Commission Consultative de
Transfusion Sanguine
blood transfusions
AIDS involuntary risk-taking through,
50–51
arm-to-arm, 19, 19n.1
France 1952 law on, 22
France professional blood donations, 19n.2
hepatitis from, 31, 31n.23, 33–34,
33–34n.26, 161, 183, 205–6
liability for, 30–31, 40–41
patient injury from toxic blood, 31,
31n.23, 32–33
U.S. on blood as service and, 31, 186–87
WWII process of, 19
Bove, Joseph, 69–70, 101–2
BPAC. See Blood Products Advisory
Committee

Carpenter, Daniel, 101
Casteret, Anne-Marie, 2–3, 45–46,
112n.17, 125
blood system attack by, 83
CNTS 1985 meeting record, 2–3, 2n.3,
84–85, 84n.12
on government betrayal, 83–84
Nau on, 83
on scandal of contaminated blood, 83
causal stories (Stone) of HIV/blood
contamination, 15–16, 108–10, 129–30,
141, 141nn.1–2, 177–78
CBER. See Center for Biologics Evaluation
and Research

CCBC. See Council of Community Blood
Centers
CCTS. See Commission Consultative de
Transfusion Sanguine
CDC. See Centers for Disease Control
Center for Biologics Evaluation and
Research (CBER), of FDA, 37–38,
100
Centers for Disease Control (CDC),
70–71, 192–93
AABB, ARC, CCBC and ABRA
meetings with, 64–65, 64n.34
accusations against, 66–67, 69–70,
101–2
on AIDS threat to blood supply, 62–64
Atlanta January 1983 meeting, 62–63,
65–66, 66n.36, 101–2
blood industry meetings, 64–65, 64n.34
dominance of AIDS epidemic
identification and communication
by, 61–62
EIS of, 63–64
FDA meetings with, 62n.30
French Working Group on AIDS and,
62–63, 67
French Working Group partnering
with, 67
on HIV contamination of blood supply
probability, 37n.35, 54
interconnected relationships in blood
field, 63–65, 64n.35
lack of authority and autonomy, 71–72
on mandatory high-risk donors
deferral, 68, 73–74
MMWR report on hemophiliacs PCP,
63, 184
PHS, FDA, NIH, NHF crisis, dismissal
of, 67–68
Reagan administration and budget
constraints, 71–72
scientific uncertainty, 69, 71
U.S and blood crisis 1981-1985, 62–69
Centre National de Transfusion Sanguine
(CNTS) (National Blood Transfusion
Center). See also Soulier
ADP litigation, target of, 110
AFH relationship with, 85n.15, 103,
183–84